Manual of Sperm Retrieval and Preparation in Human Assisted Reproduction

Cambridge Laboratory Manuals in Assisted Reproductive Technology

Titles in the series:

Manual of Sperm Retrieval and Preparation in Human Assisted Reproduction

Edited by

Ashok Agarwal
The Cleveland Clinic Foundation, Cleveland, OH, USA

Ahmad Majzoub
Hamad Medical Corporation, Doha, Qatar

Sandro C. Esteves
ANDROFERT - Andrology & Human Reproduction Clinic, and University of Campinas (UNICAMP),
Campinas, Brazil

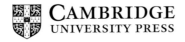

CAMBRIDGE
UNIVERSITY PRESS

CAMBRIDGE
UNIVERSITY PRESS

University Printing House, Cambridge CB2 8BS, United Kingdom

One Liberty Plaza, 20th Floor, New York, NY 10006, USA

477 Williamstown Road, Port Melbourne, VIC 3207, Australia

314–321, 3rd Floor, Plot 3, Splendor Forum, Jasola District Centre, New Delhi – 110025, India

79 Anson Road, #06–04/06, Singapore 079906

Cambridge University Press is part of the University of Cambridge.

It furthers the University's mission by disseminating knowledge in the pursuit of education, learning, and research at the highest international levels of excellence.

www.cambridge.org
Information on this title: www.cambridge.org/9781108792158
DOI: 10.1017/9781108867245

First published 2021

Printed in Singapore by Markono Print Media Pte Ltd

A catalogue record for this publication is available from the British Library.

ISBN 978-1-108-79215-8 Paperback

To my father Professor RC Agarwal (late) for instilling the virtues of honesty, dedication, and hard work. To my wonderful wife, Meenu, sons, Rishi and Neil-Yogi, for their unconditional love and support. To Professor Kevin Loughlin (Harvard Medical School), Professor Anthony Thomas (late) (Cleveland Clinic), and Professor Edmund Sabanegh (Cleveland Clinic) for their friendship, guidance, and support, and for making an indelible positive impression on my life. To my associates at work, large number of researchers and students, and most importantly the patients who placed their trust in our work.

Ashok Agarwal

I would like to dedicate this book to my wife, Zeinab, and our two lovely daughters, Sarah and Tala, for their love and support; to my mentors, Dr. Edmund Sabanegh and Professor Ashok Agarwal (Cleveland Clinic), for their guidance and support and for all the opportunities they made possible.

Ahmad Majzoub

To my father, Waldemar Esteves (late), for instilling the virtues of integrity, perseverance, and enthusiasm. To my wife, Fabiola, my sons, Alexandre and Catarina, for their devotion, love, and support. To my team at ANDROFERT Clinic for their unconditional support and hard work. To my mentors Professor Nelson Rodrigues Netto Jr. (late) (UNICAMP), Dr. Anthony Thomas Jr. (late) (Cleveland Clinic), Professor Agnaldo Cedenho (Federal University of São Paulo), and Dr. Ashok Agarwal (Cleveland Clinic) for their guidance, support, and for being giants who take their apprentices by their hands and teach them how to climb; once on their shoulders, you have shown us what to see . . . helping us to see better and farther. To my colleague Dr. Ahmad Majzoub for sharing the enthusiasm in the study and practice of andrology and male infertility. And lastly, to all my patients who put their trust in my work and from whom I learn more and more daily.

Sandro C. Esteves

Contents

Contributors

Mohamed Adnan
Department of Urology, Tulane University,
New Orleans, Louisiana, USA

Daniela Paes de Almeida Ferreira Braga
Fertility Medical Group – São Paulo,
Brazil
Sapientiae Insitute – São Paulo, Brazil

Ashok Agarwal
Andrology Center, Department of Urology,
American Center for Reproductive Medicine,
Cleveland Clinic, Cleveland,
OH, USA

Jason P. Akerman
University of North Carolina, Department of
Urology, Chapel Hill, NC, USA

Ahmed H. Almalki
Urology Department, Hamad Medical Corporation,
Doha, Qatar

Laith M. Alzweri
Department of Urology, University of Texas Medical
branch, Galveston Texas, USA

Catalina Barbarosie
American Center for Reproductive Medicine,
Cleveland Clinic, Cleveland, OH, USA
Faculty of Biology, University of Bucharest,
Bucharest, Romania

Edson Borges
Fertility Medical Group – São Paulo, Brazil
Sapientiae Insitute – São Paulo, Brazil

Darren J. Bryk
Department of Urology, Glickman Urological and
Kidney Institute, Cleveland Clinic Foundation,
Cleveland, OH, USA

Chak-Lam Cho
Department of Surgery, Union Hospital, Shatin,
Hong Kong

Gianmartin Cito
Department of Urology, Careggi Hospital, University
of Florence, Florence, Italy

Jordan A. Cohen
Department of Urology, University of Miami, Miami,
FL, USA

R. Matthew Coward
UNC Fertility, Raleigh, NC, USA

Sandro C. Esteves
ANDROFERT, Andrology & Human Reproduction
Clinic, Campinas, Brazil
Department of Surgery (Division of Urology),
University of Campinas (UNICAMP), Campinas,
Brazil
Faculty of Health, Department of Clinical Sciences,
Aarhus University, Aarhus, Denmark

Kareim Khalafalla
Urology Department, Hamad Medical corporation,
Doha, Qatar

Manesh Kumar Panner Selvam
American Center for Reproductive Medicine,
Cleveland Clinic, Cleveland, OH, USA

Neel V. Parekh
Department of Urology, Glickman Urological and
Kidney Institute, Cleveland Clinic Foundation,
Cleveland, OH, USA

Ahmad Majzoub
Department of Urology, Hamad Medical
Corporation, Doha, Qatar
Weill Cornell Medicine – Qatar, Doha, Qatar

Kruyanshi Master
American Center for Reproductive Medicine,
Cleveland Clinic, Cleveland, OH, USA

Omer Raheem
Department of Urology, Tulane University,
New Orleans, Louisiana, USA

Ranjith Ramasamy
Department of Urology, University of Miami,
FL, USA

Ryan Scribner
Memorial Medical Center, Springfield, IL, USA

Rupin Shah
Lilavati Hospital & Research Centre, Mumbai, India

Rakesh Sharma
American Center for Reproductive Medicine,
Cleveland Clinic, Cleveland, OH, USA

Amanda Souza Setti
Fertility Medical Group – São Paulo, Brazil
Sapientiae Insitute – São Paulo, Brazil

Nick N. Tadros
Department of Surgery, SIU School of Medicine,
Springfield, IL, USA

Sarah C. Vij
Department of Urology, Glickman Urological and
Kidney Institute, Cleveland Clinic Foundation,
Cleveland, OH, USA

Editor Biographies

Dr. Ashok Agarwal is the Head of Andrology Center and Director of Research at the American Center for Reproductive Medicine. He holds these positions at the Cleveland Clinic Foundation, where he is Professor of Surgery (Urology) at the Lerner College of Medicine of Case Western Reserve University. Ashok was trained in male infertility and andrology at the Brigham and Women's Hospital and Harvard Medical School, and has over 28 years of experience in directing busy male infertility diagnostic and fertility preservation services. He is an editor of over 40 medical textbooks on male infertility, ART, fertility preservation, DNA damage, and antioxidants.

Dr. Majzoub is a consultant at the Department of Urology and Program Director of the Andrology and Male Infertility Fellowship at Hamad Medical Corporation, Doha, Qatar. He is an Arab Board Certified Urologist and has undergone Clinical and Research Fellowship in Andrology at the world-famous Glickman Urological and Kidney Institute and the American Center for Reproductive Medicine at Cleveland Clinic Foundation, Cleveland, USA.

Dr. Majzoub is actively involved in the field of medical research, with over 150 research publications in peer-reviewed journals and several book chapters mainly focusing on andrology and men's health. He has also co-edited several books and special issues on various aspects of male infertility.

Dr. Sandro C. Esteves is Medical Director of ANDROFERT, a referral fertility center for male reproduction in Brazil. Dr. Esteves is also Collaborating Professor in the Department of Surgery (Division of Urology) at the University of Campinas (UNICAMP, Brazil) and Honorary Professor of Reproductive Endocrinology at the Faculty of Health, Aarhus University, Denmark. Professor Esteves has published over 300 peer-reviewed scientific papers, authored over 80 book chapters, and served as an editor of 10 textbooks related to male infertility and assisted reproductive technology. He serves on the editorial board of several journals and is Associate Editor of *International Brazilian Journal of Urology* and *Frontiers in Endocrinology (Reproduction)*.

Preface

The field of male infertility has witnessed major clinical advancements in recent years, and perhaps the most important of these was the development of testicular sperm retrieval procedures that allowed men with azoospermia to father their biological children. Epididymal sperm retrieval procedures were first performed in the 1980s for men with obstructive azoospermia. The realization that men with nonobstructive azoospermia may indeed have focal areas of testicular sperm production together with the documented fertilizing ability of testicular spermatozoa allowed the development of testicular sperm retrieval procedures in the 1990s. Subsequently, testicular sperm retrieval underwent further refinement with the introduction of microsurgery, which improved the sperm retrieval rate and at the same time reduced the potential adverse impact of surgery on testicular parenchyma. Extensive research has been conducted in attempts to study the predictors of positive sperm retrieval, hoping to increase the outcome of surgical sperm retrieval procedures.

This manual presents recent advancements in the surgical management of azoospermia patients. It is divided into three parts: Part I serves as an introduction presenting important anatomic and physiologic aspects of the reproductive tract and demonstrating the ideal methods for evaluating candidates of sperm retrieval. Part II elaborates on the surgical techniques of sperm retrieval in a variety of clinical scenarios. Moreover, it investigates the predictors of successful sperm retrieval and explores methods for enhancing sperm retrieval outcomes. Finally, Part III focuses on the laboratory handling of retrieved sperm and sperm cryopreservation, and explores future directions aimed at optimizing embryologists' work in the lab.

We are confident that our book will be a useful guide for reproductive surgeons, IVF specialists, embryologists, and other healthcare workers practicing reproductive medicine. In addition, it will be a valuable resource for students and researchers wishing to learn more about this subject. We are greatly thankful to large number of experts who worked hard to contribute the latest, well written, and well researched articles; this book would not be possible without their active support. We wish to express our deep gratitude to the superb organizational and management skills of Camille Lee-Own, publishing assistant at Cambridge University Press, and the overall support and supervision of this project by Nick Dunton, publisher at Cambridge University Press. This book is dedicated to our parents, families, mentors, and patients.

Editors:
Professor Ashok Agarwal, Cleveland Clinic, USA
Dr. Ahmad Majzoub, Hamad Medical Corporation, Qatar
Professor Sandro Esteves, Androfert, Brazil

Anatomy and Physiology of the Male Reproductive System

Ryan T. Scribner and Nicholas N. Tadros

The male reproductive system is an incredibly complex yet balanced network of central nervous system circuits and internal and external pelvic organs. The feedback circuit composed of the hypothalamic–pituitary–gonadal (HPG) axis leads to reproductive tract formation and development during embryogenesis, sexual maturation at puberty, and testosterone and sperm production by the testis. The HPG axis continues to stimulate androgen production throughout adulthood to maintain adequate testosterone and sperm production. This axis and the internal and external pelvic organs are the key components in the male reproductive system. This chapter outlines the anatomy and physiology of the male reproductive system, including the

HPG axis, control of testosterone production and spermatogenesis within the testis, maturation of sperm within the epididymis, and the transportation of sperm from the distal epididymis through the ejaculatory duct during seminal emission (Figure 1.1).

1.1 Hypothalamic–Pituitary–Gonadal Axis

1.1.1 Basic Hormone and Feedback Concepts

The HPG axis plays an essential role in development, sexual maturation, and maintenance of the male

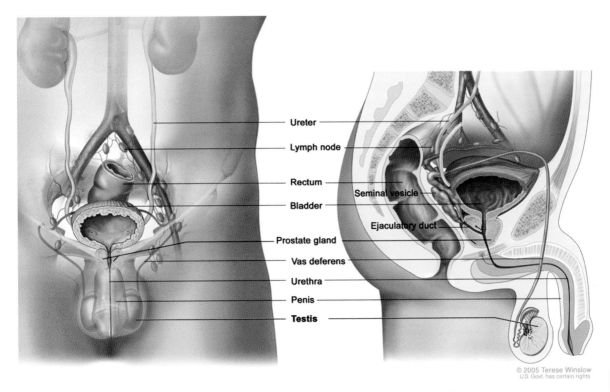

Ureter
Lymph node
Rectum
Seminal vesicle
Bladder
Ejaculatory duct
Prostate gland
Vas deferens
Urethra
Penis
Testis

Figure 1.1 Anatomy of the male reproductive and urinary systems. Reprinted by permission of Terese Winslow

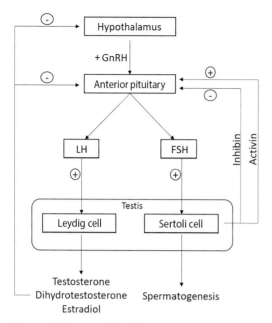

Figure 1.2 Diagram of the HPG axis in males. +, positive feedback; −, negative feedback.

reproductive system. The hypothalamus, anterior pituitary, and gonads each secrete hormones necessary for communication between the individual components of this axis (Figure 1.2). The hormones secreted by the HPG axis come in two flavors: peptide and steroid hormones. Peptide hormones are small, hydrophilic proteins that are unable to cross the plasma membrane; they exert their effects via cell surface receptors and signal transduction. Examples of peptide hormones include gonadotropin-releasing hormone (GnRH), follicle-stimulating hormone (FSH), and luteinizing hormone (LH). Steroid hormones are lipophilic hormones derived from cholesterol that are able to freely diffuse across the plasma membrane and bind to intracellular receptors in the cytoplasm and nucleus. This steroid hormone–receptor complex is able to bind directly to DNA and operate as a transcription factor for gene expression. Examples of peptide hormones include estrogen and testosterone.

1.1.2 Components of the Reproductive Axis

1.1.2.1 Hypothalamus

The hypothalamus is connected to a variety of areas in the central nervous system and has many functions. The most notable function of the hypothalamus

is its central neuroendocrine function, and its main role in the HPG axis is to transport hormones to the anterior pituitary for stimulation of peptide hormone release and gonadal regulation. Gonadotropin-releasing hormone is the most important hypothalamic hormone for reproduction. It is a 10-amino acid neuropeptide hormone produced by hypothalamic neurosecretory cells. It is released in a pulsatile manner into the hypophyseal portal circulation, where it is delivered directly to the anterior pituitary gland and stimulates LH and FSH production and secretion [1]. When GnRH pulses do not occur at the appropriate amplitude or frequency, possible complications include hypogonadism and decreased plasma gonadotropins.

1.1.2.2 Anterior Pituitary

The anterior pituitary is the target site of GnRH released from the hypothalamus, and stimulation of the anterior pituitary by GnRH results in production and release of adenohypophyseal hormones. Release of LH and FSH from the anterior pituitary is essential for regulation of testicular function. Both LH and FSH are released in a pulsatile manner, and negative feedback from estrogen and testosterone affect the secretion of these hormones by the anterior pituitary. In the testis, LH acts on Leydig cells to stimulate the production of testosterone, whereas FSH acts on Sertoli cells within the seminiferous tubules to initiate spermatogenesis during puberty and maintain spermatogenesis throughout adulthood.

1.1.2.3 Testis

The human testis is essential in steroidogenesis and the production of spermatozoa. Once LH acts on the Leydig cells and testosterone is produced, the active testosterone metabolites dihydrotestosterone and estradiol are formed to act on target organs. After FSH acts on Sertoli cells, various proteins and growth factors are produced, leading to seminiferous tubule growth during development and sperm production at puberty. The testis also produces other regulatory proteins such as inhibin and activin. Inhibin is produced by the Sertoli cells in response to FSH stimulation, acting as a negative feedback inhibitor at the anterior pituitary, whereas activin has a stimulatory effect on FSH production [2]. Testosterone and estrogen are also capable of regulating hormone production via feedback suppression on the hypothalamus and anterior pituitary.

1.2 The Testis

1.2.1 Testis Structure and Function

1.2.1.1 Testicular Parenchyma

The human testis is an external, ovoid organ that hangs from the inguinal canal by the spermatic cord and is located within the scrotum. Each testis has a volume of 15–30 ml and measures 3.5–5.5 cm in length by 2.0–3.0 cm in width [3]. Each testis contains two compartments: an interstitial compartment made up of Leydig cells that are responsible for testosterone production and secretion, and a seminiferous tubule compartment that is made up of Sertoli cells and germ cells, where spermatogenesis occurs. Approximately 80 percent of testicular volume is dedicated to spermatogenesis. Figure 1.3 represents a lateral cross-section view of the human testis.

1.2.1.2 Testicular Vascular Supply and Innervation

Arterial blood supply to the testis originates from three sources: the testicular artery, which arises from the abdominal aorta; the cremasteric artery, which arises from the inferior epigastric artery; and the deferential artery, which arises from the superior or inferior vesical arteries. The pampiniform plexus is an intricate venous network responsible for venous return from the testes to the testicular vein and temperature regulation of the testis. It is this counter-current heat exchange that is necessary for maintaining a testicular temperature lower than normal body temperature that is ideal for sperm maturation. The testis is innervated by the intermesenteric nerves and renal plexus [2].

1.2.1.3 Interstitium

The main component of the testis interstitium is Leydig cells, which are responsible for testicular androgen production. Cholesterol is the precursor to testosterone synthesis within the Leydig cells and undergoes several enzymatic reactions once inside the cells to be converted into testosterone. Regulation of androgen synthesis is controlled by numerous factors. The feed-forward mechanism of testosterone synthesis involves hypothalamic GnRH stimulation of the anterior pituitary, which leads to LH release and activation of testosterone production in Leydig cells. The other important regulatory mechanism of testosterone synthesis is via negative feedback of peptide and steroid hormones produced by

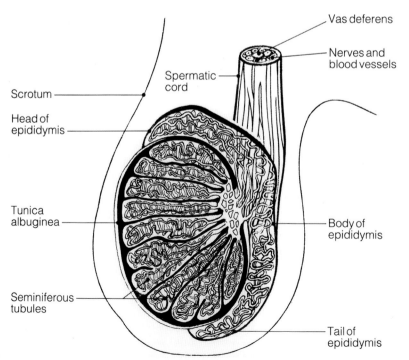

Figure 1.3 Lateral cross-section view of a human testis. Courtesy of the National Cancer Institute

the testis. Testosterone and estradiol act at the hypothalamus and the anterior pituitary to inhibit GnRH and gonadotropin secretion [3].

1.2.1.4 Seminiferous Tubules

The seminiferous tubule compartment of the testis is composed of Sertoli cells and germ cells, where spermatogenesis occurs. Sertoli cells have many functions, most of which are associated with germ cell development and movement. The following are some of the most important functions of Sertoli cells: (1) provide structural support; (2) create tight junctions that form an immunological blood–testis barrier; (3) contribute to germ cell migration and spermiation; and (4) nourish germ cells via secretory products [4].

Germ cells are located within the seminiferous tubules of the testis and give rise to spermatozoa for male reproduction. Germ cell lines are established by week four of embryogenesis, and somatic cells surrounding the germ cells lead to germ cell differentiation into the male or female pathway. In males, these somatic cells that lead to germ cell differentiation are the Sertoli and Leydig cells. Once directed down the male path, the gonocytes migrate to the basal membrane and become spermatogonia around six months after birth, remaining dormant until puberty [5].

Surrounding the seminiferous tubules are multiple layers of tissue, called peritubular tissue, which contains peritubular myoid cells that are thought to have various functions within the testis. Peritubular myoid cells are believed to create a smooth muscle layer surrounding the tubules that exerts a contractile force to traffic spermatozoa throughout the testis. In addition, myoid cells within the peritubular tissue are also responsible for maintaining spermatogonial stem cells. Studies have shown that peritubular myoid cells secrete GDNF (glial cell derived neurotrophic factor) during spermatogenesis, leading to signaling of a co-receptor RET, which leads to upregulation in Src family kinase (SFK) signaling and eventually self-renewal of spermatogonial stem cells via activation of genes encoding transcription factors [6]. Knockout studies of the GDNF pathway have demonstrated loss of spermatogonia and infertility, and overexpression studies of GDNF have revealed buildup of spermatogonial stem cells with no differentiation, leading to the conclusion that GDNF signaling is crucial for maintaining spermatogonial stem cells [6].

The blood–testis barrier is the barrier between the seminiferous tubules and the blood vessels within the testis. This barrier is actually composed of the Sertoli cells of the seminiferous tubules, which is why it is also referred to as the Sertoli cell barrier. The blood–testis barrier is composed of four separate cell junctions – tight junctions, ectoplasmic specializations, desmosomes, and gap junctions – which are all present between Sertoli cells and create two separate compartments within the blood–testis barrier: the basal and adluminal compartments [7]. This allows germ cells to be isolated from blood vessels and the lymphatic systems within the adluminal compartment, creating a microenvironment necessary for the completion of meiosis without a normal immune response from the male's immune system acting against the newly created sperm [7].

1.2.2 Spermatogenesis

Spermatogenesis is the process by which spermatozoa are produced from germ cells within the seminiferous tubules of the testis. This process takes place at puberty and continues throughout adulthood. Spermatogenesis in humans occurs in three stages: (1) a mitotic phase known as spermatocytogenesis in which stem cells divide to produce Type A spermatogonia that replace themselves or Type B spermatogonia that go down the differentiation path into spermatozoa; (2) a meiotic phase in which primary spermatocytes undergo division to produce haploid spermatids; and (3) a metamorphic phase known as spermiogenesis in which spermatids become spermatozoa. As mentioned previously, it is believed that Sertoli cells are responsible for structural support and germ cell nourishment throughout spermatogenesis. The entire process takes approximately 74 days to complete and happens at different times in different parts of the testis. This creates an overlapping production cycle in which spermatogonia can be found at different states of maturation throughout the testis.

1.2.2.1 Testis Stem Cells

In order for normal spermatogenesis to occur, testis stem cells must migrate correctly during embryogenesis, undergo renewal to replace themselves during spermatocytogenesis, and proliferate to produce daughter cell lines capable of forming mature spermatozoa. Gonocytes migrate and become spermatogonia around six months of age, remaining dormant until puberty. Once puberty occurs, mitotic division results in two separate cell lines, and GDNF secretion during spermatogenesis aids in the maintenance of spermatogonial stem cells. These separate cell lines lead to the proliferation of Type A spermatogonia that replenish themselves, or Type B spermatogonia that differentiate into spermatozoa.

1.2.2.2 Meiosis

Meiosis consists of a first and second cellular division, during which primary and secondary spermatocytes are produced, respectively. When normal spermatogonia first enter meiosis, their karyotype is originally 46,XY; however, after the second cellular division and completion of meiosis, haploid spermatids are produced containing a 23,X or 23,Y karyotype. This entire process from Type B spermatogonia to haploid spermatids last approximately 24 days in humans, and adjacent spermatocytes remain attached to one another via cytoplasmic bridges to allow for the sharing of mRNA and coordinated progression throughout meiosis [8]. Genetic recombination occurs during the pairing of homologous chromosomes in prophase, allowing for the exchange of DNA between maternal and paternal homologues, which results in genetic variation in subsequent generations.

1.2.2.3 Spermiogenesis

Throughout spermiogenesis, the spermatids produced during meiosis undergo various changes to mature into spermatozoa. The sperm head is reshaped, DNA undergoes condensation, cytoplasm is reduced, the acrosome is formed from the Golgi complex, and the axoneme is formed from centrioles and continues to grow [8]. At the end of spermiogenesis, mature spermatozoa are eventually released from the Sertoli cells into the seminiferous tubule lumen in a process known as spermiation.

1.3 The Epididymis

1.3.1 Epididymal Structure

The epididymis is the transport duct for spermatozoa between the testis and vas deferens. It is divided into three parts: a head (caput), a body (corpus), and a tail (cauda). As sperm travel throughout the epididymis, they undergo final maturation processes allowing for increased motility and fertility.

1.3.1.1 Vascular Supply and Innervation

The head and body of the epididymis both receive blood supply from a branch of the testicular artery, whereas the tail of the epididymis is supplied by the deferential artery of the vas. The epididymis is innervated by the intermediate spermatic nerve, which arises from the superior portion of the hypogastric plexus, and inferior spermatic nerve, which is a branch of the pelvic plexus [2].

1.3.1.2 Epididymal Epithelium

The epithelium of the epididymal tubule consists of principal, basal, apical, and clear cells [9]. Principal and basal cells make up the majority of the epididymal tubule cells, and the principal cells with their long stereocilia are responsible for resorption of testicular fluid and secretion of nutrients for sperm maturation. The basal cells are located at the base of principal cells and are undifferentiated precursors of principal cells. Apical and clear cells are the remaining groups of cells found within the epididymal epithelium. Apical cells are more commonly found within the head of the epididymis and contain an abundance of mitochondria, whereas the clear cells are more commonly found within the tail and contain a large number of endocytic vesicles and lipid droplets [9].

1.3.1.3 Epididymal Contractile Tissue

Just as there is a smooth muscle layer surrounding the seminiferous tubules to traffic spermatozoa throughout the testis, similar contractile tissue surrounds the epididymis. As a sperm traverses from the head to the tail of the epididymis, the amount of smooth muscle surrounding the epididymal tubule increases along its course. This allows for increased peristalsis to advance the sperm along the length of the epididymis toward the vas deferens.

1.3.2 Epididymal Function

Aside from serving as the transport system for spermatozoa between the testis and vas deferens, the epididymis also has two other functions: (1) to act as a reservoir for sperm storage during the process of spermatogenesis; and (2) to assist in sperm maturation and promote increased motility and fertility via several biochemical changes.

1.3.2.1 Sperm Transport

It has been estimated that sperm transport through the human epididymis ranges anywhere from 2 to 12 days, and this transport time is independent of a male's age [10]. Prior to Johnson and Varner's studies, it was thought that humans had delayed epididymal transit times to accommodate for the slow process of spermatogenesis and sperm maturation; however, Johnson and Varner's research contested these claims and showed that men with greater rates of daily spermatozoan production have faster epididymal transit times, with some having a transit time of just two days, indicating maturation may occur very rapidly within the epididymis [10].

1.3.2.2 Sperm Storage

After sperm traverse through the head and body of the epididymis, a large majority are retained in the tail for storage. Several findings support the fact that the caudal epididymis is the spermatozoa storage site: (1) following repeated ejaculation, sperm were expelled from the caudal epididymis, but the rate of sperm transit throughout the caput and corpus remain unchanged; (2) the ducts proximal to the cauda epididymis have neuromusculature that results in slow, regular contractions, whereas the cauda epididymis normally has a neuromusculature that is relatively dormant but produces nerve-mediated, short, forceful contractions; and (3) spermatozoa in the vas deferens following ejaculation return to the cauda epididymis [11]. Although the exact amount of time that sperm can remain fertile within the cauda is unknown, some studies have indicated that caudal sperm can preserve their capability of fertilizing an egg for up to three weeks, and their motility is maintained for twice as long as their ability to fertilize [11].

1.3.2.3 Sperm Maturation

As sperm pass through the epididymis, they must undergo maturation processes to increase motility and fertility. In previous studies, spermatozoa released from the caput epididymis were immotile or displayed weak, beating movements that did not result in forward movement; however, motile spermatozoa with strong, beating, forward movements were first identified in the corpus, and an even larger population was found in the cauda [12]. Some studies have questioned the claims that epididymal maturation is necessary in humans, noting that spermatozoa aspirated from the efferent ducts or from blocked ducts has led to fertilization *in vitro*, and some patients are capable of conceiving after anastomosis of the rete testis or seminiferous tubule to the vas deferens [11]. In men

with nonobstructive azoospermia, finding sperm within the testis during a procedure known as testicular sperm extraction allows those sperm to be used for *in vitro* fertilization (IVF) with intracytoplasmic sperm injection, further questioning the need for epididymal maturation, at least in the artificial setting of IVF. The maturation mechanisms for gaining motility may be extraordinarily different when comparing normal physiological conditions versus abnormal tract conditions. In addition to gaining motility, sperm must undergo changes that increase their ability to fertilize an oocyte. *In vivo* and *in vitro* studies have yet to show that testicular spermatozoa are capable of fertilizing an oocyte, and additional reports show that spermatozoa must pass through a proximal portion of the epididymis in order to bind the zona pellucida and penetrate the oocyte [11]. Several important biochemical changes take place that allow for better migration through the female reproductive tract and improved zona pellucida adherence: (1) the spermatozoan membrane gains a net negative charge; (2) disulfide bonds are formed in the nucleus and perinuclear matrix, leading to increased structural stability during egg penetration; and (3) exchange of glycosylated proteins and sterols in the sperm plasmalemma [12]. These maturation processes observed in the epididymis are necessary for males to achieve paternity without assisted reproductive means.

1.4 Vas Deferens

1.4.1 Vas Deferens Structure

The vas deferens is a tubular organ derived from the mesonephric duct and functions as a transport system between the epididymis and ejaculatory ducts. The vas deferens is approximately 30–35 cm long, 2–3 mm in diameter, and has a luminal diameter of 300–500 μm [9]. In cross-section, the vas deferens is composed of an outer adventitial sheath containing nerves and blood vessels, a muscular wall composed of inner and outer longitudinal and circular smooth muscle, and an inner mucosal layer composed of pseudostratified columnar epithelium with stereocilia [9]. The three-layered muscular wall gives the vas deferens the greatest muscle-to-lumen ratio compared to any other hollow organ in the human body. Its arterial blood supply is derived from the artery of the vas deferens, and the veins of the vas deferens drain into the pelvic venous plexus.

1.4.2 Vas Deferens Function

The vas deferens serves two functions in the male reproductive system: (1) transport of sperm from the epididymis to the ejaculatory ducts; and (2) absorption and secretion of various substances to create a viable environment for the sperm.

1.4.2.1 Sperm Transport

The most widely understood function of the vas is to act as a conduit for sperm between the epididymis and ejaculatory ducts. Peristaltic contractions of the thick muscular layer surrounding the vas deferens aids in this transport.

1.4.2.2 Absorption and Secretion

After complex studies of the vas deferens using light and electron microscopy, the absorptive and secretory functions of the human vas were discovered based on the epithelial morphology. Electron micrographs of principal cells discovered that these particular cells are capable of synthesizing proteins and glycoproteins, and additional studies revealed that the endocytotic invaginations of the principal cell membranes, the phagolysosomes, and the small, coated vesicles in the cytoplasm are important for protein absorption from the lumen [13]. Two other interesting findings were discovered in Hoffer's studies: (1) the presence of mitochondrion-rich cells and dense inclusion bodies in the nuclei of principal cells; and (2) mitochondrion-rich cells that appear near puberty. Although the function of these cells is still in question, it is hypothesized that the mitochondrion-rich cells are involved in the acidification of seminal plasma, and the inclusion bodies may be androgen-dependent structures within the vas deferens with an unknown function [13]. These additional discoveries have brought into question the previous belief that the vas deferens was only a transport duct for sperm.

1.5 Seminal Vesicle and Ejaculatory Ducts

1.5.1 Seminal Vesicle Structure

The seminal vesicles are paired glands located at the base of the prostate, measuring approximately 5–10 cm in length and 3–5 cm in diameter, with an average volume of 13 ml [9]. Each seminal vesicle is a coiled tube with diverticula scattered throughout its wall, and the wall of each vesicle is composed of three layers: an external connective tissue layer, a middle smooth muscle layer, and an inner mucosal layer lined with cuboidal and pseudostratified columnar epithelium and protein-secreting cells [9]. The primary blood supply of the seminal vesicles comes from the vesiculodeferential artery, which is a branch of the umbilical artery, and venous drainage occurs via the vesiculodeferential vein [14]. The seminal vesicles are innervated by parasympathetic input from the pelvic plexus, and sympathetic input from the hypogastric nerves.

1.5.2 Ejaculatory Duct Structure

The lower pole of the seminal vesicle consists of a straight duct that merges with the ampulla of the vas deferens to form the ejaculatory duct. Each ejaculatory duct is roughly 2 cm in length, extending from the base of the prostate toward its opening on the verumontanum [9]. The ejaculatory duct walls are thin and consist of three layers: an outer fibrous layer, a thin layer consisting of smooth muscle fibers, and a mucosal layer lined by columnar epithelium [9].

1.5.3 Seminal Vesicle and Ejaculatory Duct Function

Approximately 80 percent of seminal fluid is secreted by the seminal vesicles; however, this portion of the seminal fluid is rarely seen in the first ejaculate fractions, which contain high concentrations of spermatozoa and prostate secretions [2]. The fluid secreted by the seminal vesicles is yellowish in color with a neutral to alkaline pH and contains a high concentration of fructose, coagulation proteins, and prostaglandins [9]. After fluid is produced by the seminal vesicles, it progresses through the ejaculatory ducts and empties into the prostatic urethra. The exact function of this fluid is unknown, but some studies indicate that the fructose may provide a nutrient-rich environment for spermatozoa and the coagulation proteins may assist in sperm motility and suppression of immune response in the female reproductive tract [2]. Ejaculatory duct obstruction is a rare but potentially reversible cause of obstructive azoospermia.

1.6 Spermatozoa

1.6.1 Anatomy and Physiology

The spermatozoon is a motile sperm cell that joins with an ovum to form a zygote. The human spermatozoon is approximately 60 μm in length and is composed of three units: a head, a neck, and a tail [2]. The ovaloid head is approximately 4 × 3 μm, containing condensed chromatin, nucleoproteins, and an acrosomal cap with enzymes essential for oocyte fertilization [9]. The neck contains centrioles that are necessary for connection of the sperm head to the tail. The sperm tail is divided into the middle, principal, and end pieces. The middle piece of the tail comprises the axoneme, which is composed of two central microtubules that are surrounded by nine microtubule doublets (9 + 2 microtubule arrangement), and a spiral mitochondrial sheath that generates the energy necessary for motility [3]. The principal and end pieces of the tails are both surrounded by a fibrous sheath [2]. The axoneme is the most important structure necessary for sperm motility. The microtubule doublets of the axoneme are all connected by dynein, and the ATPase function of dynein in conjunction with hundreds of other enzymes and structural proteins leads to the characteristic sperm flagellar movement [2]. Defects can occur in this microtubule structure, leading to poor sperm motility and infertility issues. Primary ciliary dyskinesia is a rare autosomal recessive genetic disorder that causes defects in the action of all cilia in the body, including flagellum of sperm.

1.7 Summary

The male reproductive system is a complex balance of hormonal regulation and pelvic organs. Spermatogenesis is regulated by pulsatile secretions of GnRH, LH, and FSH and feedback regulation on the HPG axis. Mitosis, meiosis, and spermiogenesis lead to the production of immotile spermatozoa within the seminiferous tubules of the testis. During transport through the epididymis, sperm undergo maturation processes to increase motility and fertility. Sperm are transported through the ejaculatory ducts and into the urethra during ejaculation, combining with the seminal fluid that provides a nutrient-rich environment, assists in sperm motility, and suppresses the immune response in the female reproductive tract.

References

1. Kaprara A, Huhtaniemi IT. The hypothalamus–pituitary–gonad axis: tales of mice and men. *Metabolism* 2018;**86**:3–17.

2. Turek PJ. Male reproductive physiology. In Wein AJ, Kavoussi LR, Campbell MF, Walsh PC (eds.) *Campbell–Walsh Urology*. Elsevier, Philadelphia, PA, 2016, pp. 516–537.

3. Matsumoto AM, Bremner WJ. Testicular disorders. In Melmed S, Koenig R, Rosen C, et al. (eds.) *Williams Textbook of Endocrinology*. Elsevier, Philadelphia, PA, 2016, pp. 694–784.

4. Mruk DD, Cheng CY. Sertoli–Sertoli and Sertoli–germ cell interactions and their significance in germ cell movement in the seminiferous epithelium during spermatogenesis. *Endocrine Rev* 2004;25(5):747–806

5. Stukenborg JB, Kjartansdóttir KR, Reda A, et al. Male germ cell development in humans. *Hormone Res Paediatr* 2014;81:2–12.

6. Potter, SJ, DeFalco, T. Role of the testis interstitial compartment in spermatogonial stem cell function. *Reproduction* 2017;**153**(4): R151–R162.

7. Mruk DD, Cheng CY. The mammalian blood–testis barrier: its biology and regulation. *Endocrine Rev* 2015;**36** (5):564–591.

8. de Kretser DM, Loveland K, O'Bryan M. Spermatogenesis. In Jameson JL and De Groot LJ (eds.) *Endocrinology: Adult and Pediatric*. Saunders, Philadelphia, PA, 2015, pp. 2325–2353.

9. Standring, S. *Gray's Anatomy: The Anatomical Basis of Clinical Practice*. 41st edn., Elsevier, Philadelphia, PA, 2016.

10. Johnson L, Varner DD. Effect of daily spermatozoan production but not age on transit time of spermatozoa through the human epididymis. *Biol Reprod* 1988;**39**:812–817.

11. Jones RC. To store or mature spermatozoa? The primary role of the epididymis. *Int J Androl* 2002;**22**(2):57–66.

12. Bedford JM. The epididymis revisited: a personal view. *Asian J Androl* 2015;**17**:693–698.

13. Hoffer AP. The ultrastructure of the ductus deferens in man. *Biol Reprod* 1976;**14**:425–443.

14. Braithwaite JL. The arterial supply of the male urinary bladder. *Br J Urol* 1952;**24**:64–71.

Chapter

2

Evaluation of Candidates for Sperm Retrieval

Darren J. Bryk, Neel V. Parekh, and Sarah C. Vij

2.1 Introduction

Infertility can lead to significant distress for a couple. Approximately 15 percent of couples struggle with infertility, with 20 percent of these related solely to a male factor and an additional 30 percent with a male factor contribution [1]; despite the prevalence of male infertility, males use fertility services half as often as women do [2,3]. Assisted reproductive technology (ART) with intracytoplasmic sperm injection (ICSI) allows infertile couples to achieve pregnancy and to produce live births by manipulating sperm and egg *in vitro* and return the product into the female reproductive tract [4]. The process of ART requires two patients – man and woman – for its success. Urologists often work closely with female fertility specialists and/or endocrinologists to evaluate and treat an infertile couple. From the male infertility perspective, there is a variety of treatment options used – including behavioral modifications, medications, and surgical procedures – dependent on the patient's history and clinical status, with the more severe cases requiring sperm retrieval. Sperm retrieval is the process of obtaining sperm for use in ART other than from an ejaculated semen sample; depending on the etiology of a man's infertility, sperm can be retrieved with or without a surgical procedure. In this chapter, we discuss the evaluation of an infertile male patient, with a focus on candidates and indications for sperm retrieval.

2.2 History and Physical

Evaluation for male infertility is indicated when a couple is unable to achieve pregnancy within one year of unprotected intercourse, or sooner if the female partner is over the age of 35. A patient may also present with an abnormal semen analysis or chief complaint concerning for an abnormality of the reproductive tract [1]. As with any medical complaint, the first step in evaluating an infertile male is

obtaining a detailed history and performing a thorough physical exam. For the infertile couple, female partner fertility workup should be ensured [5]. Patients should be questioned regarding prior paternity, which may indicate that a man had a functioning reproductive tract at some point and may narrow the differential for etiology. Entire past medical and surgical history should be assessed, with a focus on childhood history (e.g., history of cryptorchidism, testicular torsion, pediatric hernia/hydrocele repair), sexual function (e.g., erectile and ejaculatory function and appropriately timed intercourse), and possible exposure to spermatotoxic agents or diseases (e.g., use of chemotherapeutic agent or radiation treatment, history of infection/inflammation of any area of the reproductive tract) [6,7]. Men should also be evaluated for personal or family history of genetic disorders related to male infertility, hormonal disorders that may preclude normal testicular function or sperm production, and family history of infertility. Additionally, use of exogenous hormones or endocrine modulators may affect spermatogenesis.

On physical exam, the patient should be evaluated for presence or absence of secondary sexual characteristics that may suggest hormonal disorder. On genital exam, testis size should be evaluated, as testis size reflects spermatogenesis [8]. Epididymides should be evaluated for their presence; dilation may indicate obstruction of the reproductive tract. Presence or absence of bilateral vasa deferentia should be noted; if both are absent, cystic fibrosis gene mutation is likely [9]. Scrotum should also be examined for varicocele, which is the most common correctable cause of male infertility [10]. Scrotal ultrasound can be included for difficult or suspicious scrotal/testicular exam [6]. The phallus should be evaluated for location of urethral meatus. Digital rectal exam may provide information on whether the prostate is absent or, with suspicion of ejaculatory duct obstruction, if the seminal vesicles are dilated [7].

9

2.3 Semen Analysis

Semen analysis must be obtained in all patients undergoing infertility evaluation. Results of semen analysis can be highly variable; as such, two or three specimens should be obtained separated by 2–3 weeks [1,5] with 2–5 day pretest abstinence interval prior to each semen collection.

A semen sample is analyzed for semen volume, sperm concentration in the semen, total sperm number, percentage of motile sperm, and percentage of normal morphology. Clinical reference values for these parameters have been defined by the World Health Organization (WHO) (Table 2.1) [11]. A notable weakness of the WHO reference ranges is that the semen analysis data were obtained from fertile men; while these parameters are useful for classifying men as subfertile or fertile, no parameter individually can be used to diagnose infertility [11,12].

Still, these semen parameters provide useful information. Aspermia (absence of semen/low semen volume) may indicate anejaculation (inability to ejaculate) or retrograde ejaculation (semen enters the bladder instead of moving through the urethra during orgasm).

Azoospermia, the absence of sperm in the semen, can be classified in two modes: by the location of its etiology or by the presence or absence of obstruction of the male reproductive tract. The first set of descriptions, etiologic location, uses the testis as the focus and includes pre-testicular, testicular, and post-testicular azoospermia. Pre-testicular azoospermia involves endocrine abnormalities that negatively affect testicular development and spermatogenesis leading to secondary testicular failure. Testicular azoospermia involves pathology related to the production of sperm or testosterone, or obstruction within the testis itself, also referred to as primary

testicular failure. Post-testicular azoospermia describes abnormalities of sperm delivery after the testis through the urethral meatus, which could include ejaculatory dysfunction [13]. Obstructive compared to nonobstructive azoospermia (NOA) describes obstruction of sperm passage from testis through the male reproductive tract versus testicular failure, respectively [14]. Hormonal/endocrine evaluation is recommended in azoospermic men to further delineate the etiology of infertility.

2.4 Endocrine Evaluation

Endocrine disorders are uncommon in men with normal semen parameters. An endocrine evaluation is indicated for men with oligozoospermia (low semen count) or azoospermia, impaired sexual function, or other findings suggestive of endocrine abnormality [1]. Total testosterone and follicle-stimulating hormone (FSH) levels are the minimum that should be ordered; if low total testosterone is present, confirmatory repeat total testosterone should be ordered (ensuring an early morning measurement). Since testosterone circulates in three forms – tightly bound to sex hormone binding globulin (SHBG), loosely bound to protein (most notably, albumin), and unbound – further testing should also be performed to measure the bioavailable testosterone; thus, SHBG and albumin levels should be measured. Additionally, luteinizing hormone and prolactin levels should be measured, which may aid in determination of the source of the hormonal abnormality. Estradiol measurement can also be considered, especially in the presence of gynecomastia, as an elevated level may indicate reproductive dysfunction. [1,5,15]. Table 2.2 lists clinical fertility conditions and their relationship with these hormonal levels.

2.5 Specialized Semen Tests

As previously mentioned, semen analysis results can vary from test to test and the commonly measured semen parameters may not accurately predict infertility. There are a variety of secondary tests that can be used under certain circumstances that may aid in diagnosing the presence and etiology of infertility.

Pyospermia is defined as excessive numbers of leukocytes in the ejaculate, with a threshold value of one million/ml, and may be indicative of genital tract infection or inflammation [1,16].

Table 2.1 Clinical reference values for semen analysis [11]

Parameter	Reference value
Semen volume (ml)	1.5
Sperm concentration (10^6/ml)	15
Total sperm number (10^6)	39
Sperm motility (%)	40
Normal sperm morphology (%)	4

Table 2.2 Hormone levels for clinical fertility conditions

Condition	FSH	LH	Testosterone	Prolactin
Normal spermatogenesis	Normal	Normal	Normal	Normal
Hypogonadotropic hypogonadism	Low	Low	Low	Normal
Prolactin-secreting tumor	Normal/low	Normal/low	Low	High
Hypergonadotropic hypogonadism (primary testicular failure)	High	High	Low	Normal
Post-testicular azoospermia	Normal	Normal	Normal	Normal

FSH, follicle-stimulating hormone; LH, luteinizing hormone.

Antisperm antibodies (ASA) can form when there is a disruption in the blood–testis barrier, such as after vasectomy, testis trauma, orchitis, cryptorchidism, testis cancer, or varicocele, leading to potentially decreased motility and sperm agglutination. Antisperm antibodies are typically managed with sperm retrieval for ICSI. Thus, testing for ASA is not needed if ICSI is already indicated.

The ultrastructural arrangement of the sperm tail is important for sperm motility. In disorders such as primary ciliary dyskinesia, this structure is disturbed, which can lead to immotile sperm [5].

Fragmentation of sperm DNA integrity may negatively affect fertility. Sperm DNA testing may be indicated for men with varicocele, lifestyle risk factors for infertility or unexplained infertility, recurrent pregnancy loss, or recurrent intrauterine insemination/ICSI failures. Men with infertility and high sperm DNA fragmentation tend to have lower sperm DNA fragmentation in their testicular sperm than in ejaculated sperm and may benefit from sperm retrieval to achieve a viable pregnancy [17].

2.6 Genetic Analysis

There are a variety of genetic conditions that may play a role in male infertility [18]. As such, genetic assessment may be indicated in men without a clear etiology for infertility. Men with NOA or severe oligozoospermia are at increased risk for having a genetic abnormality [1].

Genetic testing should include a karyotype to assess for chromosomal abnormalities. The most common chromosomal disorder is aneuploidy of the X chromosome – 47,XXY – also known as Klinefelter syndrome. Several other chromosomal abnormalities are known to cause infertility, but are rare. A complete karyotype is of further importance in men undergoing sperm retrieval for ICSI, as men with karyotypic abnormalities have higher risk for miscarriage or having children with chromosomal/congenital defects [6, 19].

The AZF region on the long arm of the Y chromosome is important for normal spermatogenesis. In men with NOA or severe oligozoospermia, testing for microdeletion of the Y chromosome is indicated [6]. This test can diagnose the etiology of azoospermia and predict the likelihood of success of sperm retrieval, and thus directly guide management decisions. Along the AZF region are three subregions – AZFa, AZFb, and AZFc – of which deletions distinctively affect male fertility. Microdeletion of AZFa or AZFb predicts poor outcomes from sperm retrieval, as no data have shown evidence of success in testicular sperm retrieval [18]. Therefore, surgical sperm retrieval is not recommended in men with AZFa or AZFb microdeletions. Alternatively, AZFc microdeletion, which is the most common microdeletion type, can be associated with successful sperm retrieval and successful ICSI outcomes [1,15,18]. It should be noted that all male offspring derived from patients with a Y microdeletion will inherit the same microdeletion and will be azoospermic.

Men with congenital bilateral absence of the vas deferens (CBAVD) often have mutations in the cystic fibrosis transmembrane conductance regulator (CFTR) gene, which has an association with cystic fibrosis. If a CFTR mutation is present, there is an increased risk for having offspring (male or female) with cystic fibrosis and increased risk of male offspring with CBAVD. Even if a CFTR abnormality is not found during genetic testing, there may still be a mutation that is unable to be identified. Thus, the female partners of all men with CBAVD should be tested to assess the risk of having a child with cystic fibrosis [6]. If a CFTR gene mutation is noted in either partner, the couple should be referred to genetic counseling. Intracytoplasmic sperm injection is often used for these situations to allow for preimplantation genetic testing to establish a pregnancy that is unaffected by cystic fibrosis [13,18].

2.7 Candidates for Sperm Retrieval

2.7.1 Distinguishing Azoospermia Classification

Once a complete history is obtained, a physical exam is performed, and semen analysis and endocrine evaluation are completed, the type of azoospermia can be discerned. Figure 2.1 depicts an algorithm for distinguishing the type of azoospermia and for managing each etiology of azoospermia (which will be discussed in detail in this section). Pre-testicular (nonobstructive) azoospermia, most commonly caused by hypogonadotropic hypogonadism, rarely needs sperm retrieval as medical management can often remedy the issues.

If there is evidence of testicular or post-testicular azoospermia, distinguishing if obstruction is present or absent can guide treatment and/or sperm retrieval recommendations. Follicle-stimulating hormone level and testis size can aid in determining the type of azoospermia; FSH 7.6 IU/L or less with testis long axis greater than 4.6 cm are highly likely to have obstruction, while

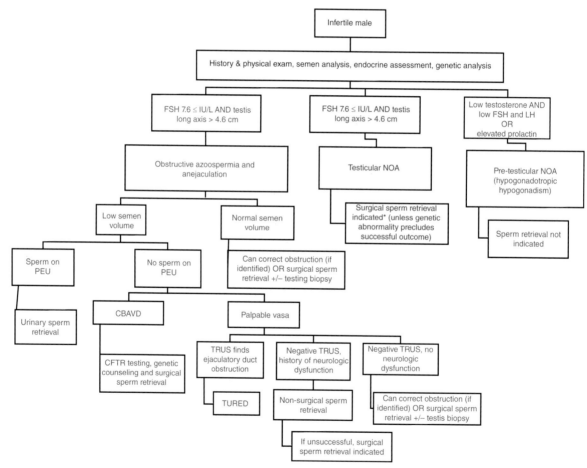

Figure 2.1 Algorithm for distinguishing the type of azoospermia and determining appropriate infertility management options.
*If clinical varicocele present, can consider varicocele repair.
FSH, follicle-stimulating hormone; LH, luteinizing hormone; NOA, nonobstructive azoospermia; PEU, post-ejaculatory urinalysis; CBAVD, congenital bilateral absence of the vas deferens; CFTR, cystic fibrosis transmembrane conductance regulator; TRUS, transrectal ultrasound; TURED, transurethral resection of the ejaculatory ducts.

FSH greater than 7.6 IU/L with testis long axis 4.6 cm or less are likely to have NOA [20].

For men with an unclear azoospermia classification, testis biopsy may be indicated. If ICSI is planned, notwithstanding the etiology of azoospermia, surgical sperm retrieval is performed and testis biopsy can be deferred. Similarly, if surgical reproductive tract reconstruction is planned, testis biopsy is usually unnecessary [13]. Still, testis biopsy can be performed, even in the aforementioned two scenarios, to obtain testicular pathology for analysis. Of note, if spermatogenesis is absent in a testis biopsy specimen, sperm can still be found in different sites of the testes during surgical sperm retrieval [5].

2.7.2 Sperm Retrieval in Nonobstructive Azoospermia

Nonobstructive azoospermia is related to spermatogenic dysfunction due to defects in the seminiferous tubules or steroidogenic dysfunction due to Leydig cell issues [5]. Regardless of the pathophysiology, if a man has NOA, surgical sperm retrieval is indicated. In men with varicocele and NOA, varicocele repair can be considered prior to surgical sperm retrieval to potentially allow for return of sperm to the ejaculate. In patients who do not have return of sperm to the ejaculate, sperm retrieval rates may be improved [21,22].

Only about 50 percent of patients with NOA will have sperm found on surgical sperm retrieval [6,19]. Still, it can be helpful for fertility prognosis if an etiology of NOA is found. If a chromosomal abnormality is noted, appropriate genetic counseling can be provided prior to surgical sperm retrieval, as there is increased risk for miscarriage and chromosomal and genetic defects [1,13]. The type of chromosomal abnormality may predict the likelihood of surgical sperm retrieval success. For Klinefelter syndrome, success rate is approximately 50 percent [23]. For a male with a karyotype 46,XX, surgical sperm retrieval is not recommended [24]. If a Y chromosome microdeletion is found, attempts at surgical sperm retrieval may only be beneficial for AZFc microdeletions and should be avoided if AZFa or AZFb microdeletions are present.

2.7.3 Sperm Retrieval in Obstructive Azoospermia and Anejaculation

While NOA tends to be associated with testicular dysfunction, which requires surgical sperm retrieval often

regardless of the pathophysiology, the management of obstructive azoospermia and anejaculation is typically based on its etiology. For these men, it is important to determine the site of obstruction, if one exists. Patients with obstructive azoospermia may be managed with correction of the obstruction if it can be identified.

During evaluation, physical exam can confirm the presence or absence of the vasa deferentia. In men with low ejaculate volume, a post-ejaculatory urinalysis (PEU) should be performed; presence of sperm in the urine suggests retrograde ejaculation rather than obstruction. While there are medications that can be used to treat this issue, commonly urinary sperm retrieval can be performed to isolate sperm for use in ART [25]. If there is no sperm in the PEU, a transrectal ultrasound should be performed to rule out ejaculatory duct obstruction [13]. If the transrectal ultrasound demonstrates dilated seminal vesicles and ejaculatory ducts, transurethral resection of the ejaculatory ducts can be performed. If the transrectal ultrasound is normal, the obstruction is likely more proximal, along the vasa deferentia and epididymides.

There are scenarios in which sperm retrieval is indicated in the presence of obstructive azoospermia. In a man with CBAVD who has undergone CFTR testing, as well as genetic counseling if needed, and desires fertility, surgical sperm retrieval is indicated. In men with hormonal profile and physical exam consistent with obstructive azoospermia but no history of reproductive tract injury and no discernable obstruction, surgical sperm retrieval may be required. Similarly, men who remain azoospermic after microsurgical vasal or epididymal reconstruction will likely require surgical sperm retrieval [19,26]. Lastly, men with known obstruction of the reproductive tract who prefer a less invasive procedure may opt for surgical sperm retrieval with vasal or epididymal sperm aspiration [14].

If no obstruction is noted and there is evidence of a neurological disorder (e.g., peripheral neuropathy or spinal cord injury), non-surgical sperm retrieval can be performed with penile vibratory stimulation or electroejaculation. If there is no evidence of anejaculation or these techniques are unsuccessful, surgical sperm retrieval may be indicated [25].

2.7.4 Sperm Retrieval for Non-Azoospermic Men

If oligozoospermia (low sperm count), teratozoospermia (abnormal sperm morphology), or asthenozoospermia (reduced sperm motility) are present, often semen from an ejaculated sample can be used for ART, with either intrauterine insemination or ICSI [27]. In men with increased sperm DNA fragmentation, ICSI outcomes may be impaired using ejaculated sperm. Infertile men without azoospermia but with high sperm DNA fragmentation may benefit from surgical sperm retrieval as testicular sperm has decreased DNA fragmentation compared to ejaculated sperm [28].

2.7.5 Considerations during Sperm Retrieval

There are many techniques for surgical sperm retrieval; descriptions of each technique are beyond the scope of this chapter. Though there is insufficient randomized control trial data to support one technique over another [29], microdissection testicular sperm extraction, which uses a microscope to examine exposed seminiferous tubules in search of active spermatogenesis, can increase sperm retrieval rates compared to open testicular sperm extraction [14,19]. During this procedure, testis histology can be evaluated to assess whether germ cells are present; testis histopathology (e.g., hypospermatogenesis, maturation arrest, Sertoli cell only) can predict the likelihood of successful surgical sperm retrieval. Still, successful sperm retrieval can be achieved even with severe spermatogenic dysfunction [19,30].

2.8 Conclusion

The evaluation of an infertile male to assess for candidacy for sperm retrieval is highly dependent on the etiology of infertility. Complete history and physical exam, as well as semen analysis, endocrine evaluation, and, likely, genetic assessment will aid in delineating obstructive versus nonobstructive azoospermia and pre-testicular versus testicular versus post-testicular azoospermia. As a result of this workup, the appropriate infertility treatment or management can be determined, including those who will likely have success with sperm retrieval.

References

1. Practice Committee of the American Society for Reproductive Medicine. Diagnostic evaluation of the infertile male: a committee opinion. *Fertil Steril* 2015;103: e18–e25.

2. Chandra A, Copen CE, Stephen EH. Infertility service use in the United States: data from the National Survey of Family Growth, 1982–2010. *Natl Health Stat Report* 2014;1–21. Available from: www.ncbi.nlm.nih.gov/pubmed/24467919.

3. Pastuszak AW, Sigalos JT, Lipshultz LI. The role of the urologist in the era of in vitro fertilization-intracytoplasmic sperm injection. *Urology* 2017;103:19–26.

4. Palermo G, Joris H, Devroey P, Van Steirteghem AC. Pregnancies after intracytoplasmic injection of single spermatozoon into an oocyte. *Lancet* 1992;340:17–18.

5. Niederberger CS. Male infertility. In Wein AJ, Kavoussi LR, Partin AW, Peters CA (eds.) *Campbell Walsh Urol*, 11th edn. Elsevier, Amsterdam, 2016, pp. 556–579.e1.

6. Katz DJ, Teloken P, Shoshany O. Male infertility: the other side of the equation. *Aust Fam Physician* 2017;46:641–646.

7. Pan MM, Hockenberry MS, Kirby EW, Lipshultz LI. Male infertility diagnosis and treatment in the era of in vitro fertilization and intracytoplasmic sperm injection. *Med Clin North Am* 2018;102:337–347.

8. Patel ZP, Niederberger CS. Male factor assessment in infertility. *Med Clin North Am* 2011;95:223–234.

9. Anguiano A, Oates RD, Amos JA, et al. Congenital bilateral absence of the vas deferens: a primarily genital form of cystic fibrosis. *JAMA* 1992;267:1794–1797.

10. Choi WS, Kim SW. Current issues in varicocele management: a review. *World J Mens Health* 2013;31:12–20.

11. Cooper TG, Noonan E, Eckardstein S et al. World Health Organization reference values for human semen characteristics. *Hum Reprod Update* 2010;16:231–245.

12. Guzick DS, Overstreet JW, Factor-Litvak P, et al. Sperm morphology, motility, and concentration in fertile and infertile men. *N Engl J Med* 2001;345:1388–1393.

13. Hwang K, Smith JF, Coward RM, et al. Evaluation of the azoospermic male: a committee opinion. *Fertil Steril* 2018;109:777–782.

14. Shin DH, Turek PJ. Sperm retrieval techniques. *Nat Rev Urol* 2013;10:723–730.

15. Esteves SC, Miyaoka R, Agarwal A. An update on the clinical assessment of the infertile male. *Clinics (Sao Paulo)* 2011;66:691–700.

16. WHO. *Laboratory Manual for the Examination and Processing of Human Semen*, 5th edn., WHO, Geneva, 2010. Available from: https://apps.who .int/iris/bitstream/handle/10665/ 44261/9789241547789_ eng.pdf;jsessionid=C7110716A3 650EF69976E4C912ED8D19? sequence=1.

17. Agarwal A, Majzoub A, Esteves SC, et al. Clinical utility of sperm DNA fragmentation testing: practice recommendations based on clinical scenarios. *Transl Androl Urol* 2016;5:935–950.

18. Hamada A, Esteves S, Agarwal A. A comprehensive review of genetics and genetic testing in azoospermia. *Clinics* 2013;68:39–60.

19. Wosnitzer M, Goldstein M, Hardy MP. Review of azoospermia. *Spermatogenesis* 2014;4:e28218.

20. Schoor Ra, Elhanbly S, Niederberger CS, Ross LS. The role of testicular biopsy in the modern management of male infertility. *J Urol* 2002;167:197–200.

21. Esteves SC, Miyaoka R, Roque M, Agarwal A. Outcome of varicocele repair in men with nonobstructive azoospermia: systematic review and meta-analysis. *Asian J Androl* 2016;18:246–253.

22. Practice Committee of the American Society for Reproductive Medicine. Management of nonobstructive azoospermia: a committee opinion. *Fertil Steril* 2018;110:1239–1245.

23. Oates RD. The natural history of endocrine function and spermatogenesis in Klinefelter syndrome: what the data show. *Fertil Steril* 2012;98:266–273.

24. Terribile M, Stizzo M, Manfredi C, et al. 46,XX testicular disorder of sex development (DSD): a case report and systematic review. *Medicina (B Aires)* 2019;55:371.

25. Mehta A, Sigman M. Management of the dry ejaculate: a systematic review of aspermia and retrograde ejaculation. *Fertil Steril* 2015;104:1074–1081.

26. Practice Committee of the American Society for Reproductive Medicine and The Society for Male Reproduction and Urology. The management of obstructive azoospermia: a committee opinion. *Fertil Steril* 2019;111:873–880.

27. Tournaye H. Male factor infertility and ART. *Asian J Androl* 2012;14:103–108.

28. Esteves SC, Roque M, Bradley CK, Garrido N. Reproductive outcomes of testicular versus ejaculated sperm for intracytoplasmic sperm injection among men with high levels of DNA fragmentation in semen: systematic review and meta-analysis. *Fertil Steril* 2017;108:456–467.e1.

29. Van Peperstraten AM, Proctor ML, Johnson NP, Philipson G. Techniques for surgical retrieval of sperm prior to intracytoplasmic sperm injection (ICSI) for azoospermia. *Cochrane Database Syst Rev* 2008;16:CD002807.

30. Donoso P, Tournaye H, Devroey P. Which is the best sperm retrieval technique for non-obstructive azoospermia? A systematic review. *Hum Reprod Update* 2007;13:539–549.

Testicular Histopathology and the Role of Testis Biopsy

Gianmartin Cito

Spermatozoa retrieved from the testis of azoospermic patients are found to be as effective as ejaculated spermatozoa in intracytoplasmic sperm injection (ICSI) cycles [1]. Performing ICSI involves treatments for both partners: the male undergoes surgery for testicular sperm recovery and the female undergoes the ovarian stimulation protocol for oocyte pickup. For this reason, an unsuccessful sperm recovery procedure could have important emotional and financial implications for the infertile couple.

In this context, sperm retrieval (SR) rates for men with obstructive azoospermia (OA) are excellent (96–100 percent), whereas the reported overall SR rates for patients with nonobstructive azoospermia (NOA) are less optimal and range from 30 to 60 percent [2]. Therefore, it is important to evaluate all clinical parameters that may predict the possibility of SR, because they would be crucial for assisting surgeons and clinicians in the correct counseling of the azoospermic patient [3].

In fact, physical examination, detailed medical history, hormonal analysis, and genetic studies will help to determine the type of azoospermia [4].

However, testicular histopathology has been found to be the most reliable predictive factor for successful SR in NOA patients since the late 1990s [5]. As reported by previous authors, the histological evaluation of testicular samples is performed after staining the tissue and cell sections with hematoxylin and eosin (H&E), and examining at least 100 different sections of seminiferous tubules. The counting is performed with a $10\times$ objective lens, exposing several tubuli in one field of vision. In cases of doubt, the presence of spermatozoa is checked using a higher magnification, and counting is performed with the $25\times$ objective lens. Tubules having their majority portion in this field are scored, and the slide is then moved sideways to bring the adjacent area into the field. When coming to the edge of the biopsy, the slide is moved up to bring the structure at the bottom edge

to the top edge and scoring continued. Based on the principal histopathological pattern, testicular histology is categorized as follows: normal spermatogenesis (NS), as shown in Figure 3.1, comprising cells from all stages of spermatogenesis and an adequate number of elongated spermatids/spermatozoa; hypospermatogenesis (HYPO), in which there is a reduction in the number of spermatogenetic cells but all stages are present, as shown in Figure 3.2; maturation arrest (MA), characterized by the absence of the later

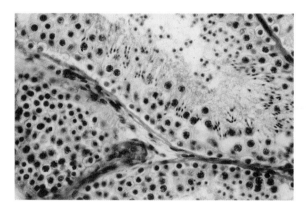

Figure 3.1 Normal spermatogenesis.

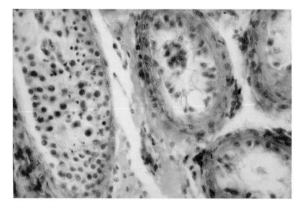

Figure 3.2 Hypospermatogenesis.

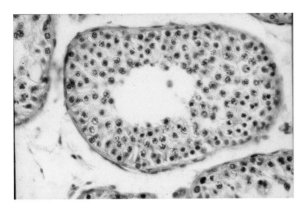

Figure 3.3 Maturation arrest.

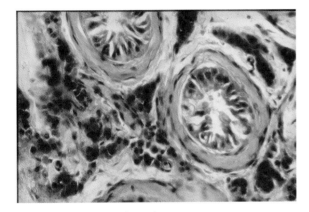

Figure 3.4 Sertoli-cell-only syndrome.

stages of spermatogenesis (Figure 3.3); Sertoli-cell-only syndrome, in which all tubules lack germ cells and are lined with Sertoli cells in the seminiferous tubules (Figure 3.4); and tubular atrophy. In addition to the registration of spermatogenesis, the number of Leydig cells is judged and recorded [6].

Follicle-stimulating hormone (FSH) concentrations and testicular volume seem to be less accurate than testicular histopathology for prediction of SR success [7]. This is supported by the fact that many patients with MA are found to have normal plasma FSH levels and testicular volume [8]. Indeed, variations in FSH concentrations can occur for reasons unrelated to spermatogenesis – FSH secretion and release are controlled by too many endocrine and paracrine factors [9]. Moreover, although the smaller testicular volume is associated with the worse possibility of SR, there is no minimum limit of testicular volume that predicts the presence of spermatozoa [10]. Previous studies also reported that higher serum

FSH concentrations were inversely related to the probability of SR in patients with NOA [11]. Indeed, FSH concentrations were inversely related to the total number of testicular germ cells; however, FSH values have poor predictive value for SR in NOA [6]. Along the same lines, the presence of associated male pathologies cannot be used as predictive factors of success [12].

The role of testicular histology as a predictor of SR has been suggested by previous several studies. Caroppo et al. showed that including the pattern of testicular histology in a model for predicting SR rates in patients with NOA improves its diagnostic accuracy [7]. Nevertheless, its application in clinical practice has been debated due to some criticism. The major and unquestionable aspect is that testicular histology may be obtained only after surgery, since a diagnostic testicular biopsy might not be a cost-effective procedure.

Based on the fact that testicular histopathology is the most accurate predictor of successful SR, some studies have proposed performing a diagnostic biopsy before assisted reproductive technologies (ARTs) [4]. In fact, the presence of elongated spermatids or spermatozoa in testicular biopsy is associated with increased SR rates [13].

However, a diagnostic biopsy itself is an invasive procedure that may have complications similar to the testicular sperm extraction (TESE) procedure, including infection, bleeding, hematoma, and tubular sclerosis [14]. This means patients undergo surgery and anesthesia twice, which increases the cost and the risk of complications. Moreover, because testicular tubules of patients with NOA are usually heterogeneous, the absence of sperm in a single biopsy does not offer assurance of a similar pattern in the entire testis. Indeed, a testicular biopsy specimen may not reflect the entire testicular tissue, bilaterally, as showed by a study that documented a 28 percent intra-individual difference in testicular histology in bilateral testicular biopsy specimens [15].

In this regard, in addition to the standard histological biopsy, previous authors have described the use of the remnants of TESE specimens after sperm has been isolated through embryological processing. In fact, only the supernatant with free sperm cells is cryopreserved or utilized for ICSI. This testicular solid tissue, defined as a "testicular pool," is waste material consisting of the residual seminiferous tubules after stretching, centrifugation, and extraction of the spermatozoa. The testicular pool has proved to be an easy-to-analyze tissue, and to be practical, manageable, and more enlightening than a single testicular biopsy for the prediction of SR and the presence of germ cell neoplasia *in situ* (GCNIS), being a tissue more representative of the entire testicular parenchyma [6].

Furthermore, when testicular histopathology shows NS, it will accurately diagnose cases of OA that were ignored clinically. However, up to 15 percent of patients with OA have an intra-testicular obstruction that is not clinically revealed [16]. It should be noted, however, that patients with OA may have some damage in spermatogenesis. It should also be noted that although patients with NOA have a serious injury of spermatogenesis, it may be possible to have areas in the testes showing foci of active NS [17]. This occurs because spermatogenesis can be very unequally distributed in a testis, which may result in a negative finding using a randomly taken testicular open biopsy. This is due to irregular distribution of spermatogenesis in testicular parenchyma, which can explain the presence of focal areas of intact spermatogenesis in patients with severe testicular atrophy. In these cases, in fact, the distribution of a minute quantity of spermatogenesis must be diffusely multi-focal.

A small diagnostic testicle biopsy specimen represents perhaps 1/1000 of the total testicular volume and possibly predicts the presence of a minute patch of spermatogenesis, according to the potential heterogeneity of testicular histopathology.

Despite these observations, another important advantage of histopathology is the revealing of GCNIS, which occurs in 1–3 percent of patients with severe male factor infertility, and which progresses to testicular cancer. Both carcinoma *in situ* and seminoma of the testis have been reported in the literature for patients undergoing TESE [18]. Banz-Jansen et al. found a tumor frequency of 1.8 percent by standard testicular biopsy in a TESE population [19].

In conclusion, testicular histopathology offers important information for counseling patients about the chances of SR success. Moreover, the results can guide clinical management in cases of failed SR, and confirm the presence of active areas or spermatogenesis on histopathology specimens. The optimal timing for the biopsy is during TESE, aiming to avoid the need for a second operation. As the pathologist analyzes the testis sample only after the surgical procedure, the histopathological pattern could guide the clinician in choosing a more suitable therapeutic option for the azoospermic patient.

References

1. Nicopoullos JD, Gilling-Smith C, Almeida PA, et al. Use of surgical sperm retrieval in azoospermic men: a meta-analysis. *Fertil Steril* 2004;82:691–701.

2. Esteves SC, Myaoka R, Orosz JE, Agarwal A. An update on sperm retrieval techniques for azoospermic males. *Clinics* 2013;68:99–110.

3. Salehi P, Derakhshan-Horeh M, Nadeali Z, et al. Factors influencing sperm retrieval following testicular sperm extraction in nonobstructive azoospermia patients. *Clin Exp Reprod Med* 2017;44(1):22–27.

4. Schlegel PN. Causes of azoospermia and their management. *Reprod Fertil Dev* 2004;16:561–572.

5. Tournaye H, Verheyen G, Nagy P, et al. Are there any predictive factors for successful testicular sperm recovery in azoospermic patients? *Hum Reprod* 1997;12:80–86.

6. Cito G, Coccia ME, Picone R, et al. Novel method of histopathological analysis after testicular sperm extraction in patients with nonobstructive and obstructive azoospermia. *Clin Exp Reprod Med* 2018;45(4):170–176.

7. Caroppo E, Colpi EM, Gazzano G, et al. Testicular histology may predict the successful sperm retrieval in patients with non-obstructive azoospermia undergoing conventional TESE: a diagnostic accuracy study. *J Assist Reprod Genet* 2017;34(1):149–154.

8. Martin-du-Pan RC, Bischof P. Increased follicle stimulating hormone in infertile men: is increased plasma FSH always due to damaged germinal epithelium? *Hum Reprod* 1995;10:1940–1945.

9. Tuttelmann F, Laan M, Grigorova M, et al. Combined effects of the variants FSHB-211G>T and FSHR 2039A>G on male reproductive parameters. *J Clin Endocrinol Metab* 2012;97:3639–3647.

10. Tsujimura A, Matsumiya K, Miyagawa Y, et al. Prediction of successful outcome of microdissection testicular sperm extraction in men with idiopathic nonobstructive azoospermia. *J Urol* 2004;172:1944–1947.

11. Colpi GM, Colpi EM, Piediferro G, et al. Microsurgical TESE versus conventional TESE for ICSI in non-obstructive azoospermia: a randomized

controlled study. *Reprod Biomed Online* 2009;18:315–319.

12. Sousa M, Cremades N, Silva J, et al. Predictive value of testicular histology in secretory azoospermic subgroups and clinical outcome after microinjection of fresh and frozen-thawed sperm and spermatids. *Hum Reprod* 2002;17:1800–1810.

13. Cissen M, Meijerink AM, D'Hauwers KW, et al. Prediction model for obtaining spermatozoa with testicular sperm extraction in men with non-obstructive azoospermia. *Hum Reprod* 2016;31(9):1934–1941.

14. Schlegel PN, Su LM. Physiological consequences of testicular sperm extraction. *Hum Reprod* 1997;12:1688–1692.

15. Plas E, Riedl CR, Engelhardt PF, Mühlbauer H, Pflüger H. Unilateral or bilateral testicular biopsy in the era of intracytoplasmic sperm injection. *J Urol* 1999;162:2010–2013.

16. Colpi GM, Pozza D. *Diagnosing Male Infertility: New Possibilities and Limits*, Karger, Basel, 1992.

17. Cito G, Coccia ME, Dabizzi S, et al. Relevance of testicular histopathology on prediction of sperm retrieval rates in case of non-obstructive and obstructive azoospermia. *Urologia* 2018;85 (2):60–67.

18. Shoshany O, Shtabholtz Y, Schreter E, et al. Predictors of spermatogenesis in radical orchiectomy specimen and potential implications for patients with testicular cancer. *Fertil Steril* 2016; 106(1):70–74.

19. Banz-Jansen C, Nikorowitsch C, Drechsler T, et al. Incidence of testicular malignancies and correlation to risk factors in a TESE population of subfertile men. *Arch Gynecol Obstet* 2012;285(1):247–253.

Chapter

4

History of Surgical Sperm Retrieval Techniques

Rupin Shah

4.1 Introduction

Operative sperm retrieval from the epididymis or testis is performed to retrieve sperm for intracytoplasmic sperm injection (ICSI) in men who have no sperm in their ejaculate. It is indicated in men with obstructive azoospermia (OA) when the obstruction is not correctable, or if the couple prefer assisted reproduction over reconstructive surgery due to social, personal, or medical reasons. It is also performed in men with nonobstructive azoospermia (NOA), since some of these men will have focal spermatogenesis in the testes, though the number of sperm in the testes is too few to appear in the ejaculate. Testicular sperm may also be used in nonazoospermic men when there is total necrozoospermia, high DNA fragmentation, cryptozoospermia, or severe oligozoospermia with recurrent *in vitro* fertilization (IVF) failure [1,2].

Surgical sperm retrieval has a long history of innovative procedures. Way back in 1955, delivering the Hunterian Lecture at the Royal College of Surgeons, Hanley described tucking a loosely folded ball of amnion under the epididymal tunica to create an artificial spermatocele and was able to recover sperm in 6 of 11 cases [3].

In the 1970s, pioneering work in creating artificial spermatoceles for sperm recovery was done by Schoysman, Wagenknecht, and Kelâmi [4]. In 1980, Cruz reported the first birth following cervical insemination with sperm recovered from a synthetic spermatocele [5], followed by another success reported by Kelâmi in 1981 [6].

However, these were anecdotal successes, and it was only after the development of IVF, and specifically ICSI, that the use of epididymal and testicular sperm became highly successful and a variety of surgical techniques were developed to recover sperm in a range of clinical situations.

4.2 Epididymal Sperm Retrieval

The first successful use of epididymal sperm for IVF was reported by Temple-Smith et al. in 1985. The patient was a man who had two failed attempts at vasectomy reversal. Using microsurgical techniques, the epididymal tubule was opened at three locations and the effluxing fluid was aspirated with a Medicut micropipette. A final concentration of 4.28 million sperm with 61 percent motility was achieved, and one of five eggs fertilized after incubation, resulting in a viable pregnancy [7].

This was soon followed by a report by Silber et al. [8] on the use of microsurgical epididymal sperm aspiration (MESA) in men with congenital vas aplasia. In his initial report, the sperm were used for IVF and fertilization rates were low. It was only after the advent of ICSI that MESA-ICSI became a very successful treatment for OA and Silber et al. reported an increase of pregnancy rates in their group of CBAVD men, from 4.5 percent with conventional IVF to 47 percent with ICSI [9].

With the increasing success and popularity of MESA-ICSI in the treatment of OA, attempts were made to simplify epididymal sperm retrieval. In 1994, at the Tenth Annual Meeting of ESHRE, Craft and colleagues presented their experience with percutaneous epididymal sperm aspiration (PESA)[10]. The procedure was quick, simple, and did not need an operating microscope. Their subsequent papers [11,12] emphasized their high success rate with the technique and PESA gained popularity.

However, many surgeons continued to prefer MESA, claiming that many more motile sperm could be retrieved and cryopreserved for multiple cycles. Accordingly, Shah [13] proposed open non-microsurgical epididymal sperm aspiration (OESA), which was a modified version of MESA that was quick, simple, did not need an operating microscope, and allowed collection of a large number of sperm under vision by puncturing the exposed epididymis with a needle and aspirating the effluxing fluid.

4.3 Testicular Sperm Retrieval

In 1993, Craft [14] reported that even testicular sperm could fertilize oocytes by IVF, but the first viable pregnancy was achieved only by the use of ICSI by Schyosman et al. [15], who performed open testicular biopsies to retrieve sperm from men with OA in whom no sperm could be retrieved from the epididymis. They used these sperm for subzonal insemination (SUZI) and ICSI, and achieved one viable pregnancy. Devroey et al. [16] confirmed that testicular sperm from men with OA were highly successful in producing viable pregnancies by ICSI. Nagy et al. [17] showed that equivalent fertilization rates could be achieved whether fresh or cryopreserved testicular sperm were used. All these preliminary studies used open, conventional testicular biopsies.

Once the fertilizing capability of sperm from normal testes was established, clinicians tried to extract and use sperm from men with testicular failure. The presence of focal areas of sperm production in testicular failure was known from earlier histological studies [18]. In 1995, Devroey et al. published their initial work on men with testicular failure and reported finding sperm by testicular sperm extraction (TESE) in 13 of 15 men [19]. Fertilization rate was 47.8 percent, and there were three ongoing pregnancies from 12 transfers. Yemini et al. [20] reported sperm in a man with tubular atrophy, while Gil-Salom et al. [21] found sperm in a man with very high FSH and a testicular histology showing Sertoli-cell-only syndrome (SCOS). In all these initial cases, testicular sperm were retrieved by conventional open biopsy, and usually multiple biopsies were required. Correlating testicular histology with sperm retrieval, Tournaye et al. [22] reported that 2.8 ± 2.5 biopsies were required in men with SCOS, and 4.5 ± 4.2 biopsies were needed in cases with maturation arrest. Accordingly, in 2004, Shah presented the SST technique in which single seminiferous tubules were pulled out through puncture holes from all over the testicular surface, thus achieving extensive random biopsies without any testicular damage [23].

Once it became clear that even men with testicular failure often had some sperm in their testes, but that this sperm production could be very localized and difficult to find, a number of different techniques for testicular sperm retrieval in NOA were developed.

Fine-needle aspiration of the testis has been in use as a diagnostic tool for over 30 years [24]. Craft et al. [12] suggested that a similar process of testicular sperm aspiration (TESA) could be used to retrieve sperm from men with OA. In 1995, Lewin et al. [25] coined the term TEFNA (testicular fine-needle aspiration) and used a 20 ml syringe mounted on an aspiration handle to perform an extensive aspiration in men with NOA. In 1999, they published their experience with 111 TEFNA procedures in 85 patients [26]. The procedure involved 15 punctures with multidirectional aspirations with a 23 G needle from each testis. They reported 48 percent sperm recovery in SCOS, 46 percent in maturation arrest, and 66 percent (four of six patients) in non-mosaic Klinefelter syndrome. Due to its ease and simplicity, TEFNA soon became a widely used alternative to open biopsies.

However, the utility of TEFNA or TESA was disputed by other clinicians. In a direct comparison of TEFNA with open biopsy in men with NOA, Friedler et al. [27] performed TEFNA (six punctures on each testis with a 21 G needle) followed by open biopsies (up to three on each side) in the same patients. TEFNA retrieved sperm in 11 percent, while sperm were found in 43 percent of the open biopsies. Even in men with OA, Tournaye et al. failed to retrieve enough sperm by TESA in 2 of 53 men.

In an attempt to improve the success of TESA, Foresta et al. [28] used a color Doppler to compare the intra-testicular blood flow patterns in men with OA and NOA. They found that spermatogenesis correlated with better blood flow and they were able to aspirate sperm in 12 of 16 testis (with no sperm on random aspiration) when the aspiration was performed in a region where blood flow was detected. Similar findings were reported by subsequent researchers [29,30].

As an alternative to fine-needle cytological aspiration, clinicians also used larger bore needles to take testicular biopsies percutaneously, obtaining tissue equivalent to an open biopsy. In 1993, Morey et al. described the use of a Biopty gun to obtain testis biopsies [31]. In 1994, Mallidis and Baker experimented with a variety of needles and concluded that the modified Menghini and Turner biopsy needles gave the best biopsy samples [32]. Other authors

[13,33] used a 19 or 18 G butterfly needle to aspirate a core of seminiferous tubules which were then pulled out of the testis to give a large percutaneous biopsy.

In 1997, Schlegel and Su reviewed their experience with conventional TESE done by multiple open biopsies or a single long biopsy and showed that these methods could cause significant testicular damage, demonstrable up to six months post-procedure [34]. Hence, they proposed microdissection TESE (mTESE) as a technique that would cause less testicular damage by taking very selective biopsies only from favorable areas that were visually identified. In 1999, Schlegel presented results in 27 men who had undergone both conventional open biopsies and mTESE biopsies on the same testes at the same session [35]. In 11/27 men (41 percent) he was able to find sperm by conventional biopsies. In an additional six men, sperm were found only in the mTESE samples, thus giving a total retrieval rate of 63 percent. Interestingly, in one case sperm were found only in the random conventional biopsies, but not in the mTESE samples from the same testis, which underscores the difficulty in visually identifying sperm-containing tubules in cases where the pattern is uniform.

These findings have been replicated by many subsequent studies, which confirm that mTESE is the most efficient method for finding sperm in NOA [36]. However, they also suggest that mTESE has an advantage only in certain testicular histologies: SCOS, testicular atrophy, and small testes with high FSH [37,38]. In cases with a visually uniform pattern of testicular parenchyma, mTESE may not be superior to random, multiple biopsies. Other studies showed that mTESE was not innocuous; Everaert et al. [39] found that 16 percent of 48 men undergoing mTESE developed *de novo* androgen deficiency. A recent meta-analysis showed that the fall in testosterone is greatest in men with Klinefelter syndrome, is maximum at 6 months, and recovers by 24 months in most, though not all, men [40].

Hence, staged sperm retrieval has been proposed [41]. During the same surgical session, progressively more invasive methods are used until sperm are found, starting with needle biopsies, progressing to therapeutic mapping, and leading up to mTESE. This helps avoid unnecessarily invasive procedures when sperm can be found by simpler methods, while ensuring that those who need mTESE are not deprived of the opportunity. While it has been suggested that such an approach may "reduce the costs, time and efforts involved in surgery" [42], this is yet to be validated in controlled studies.

An alternative approach was suggested by Shin and Turek [43], who proposed that diagnostic testicular mapping by fine-needle aspiration could be used prior to therapeutic retrieval to identify which patients would be candidates for sperm retrieval surgery, and from which areas of the testis sperm were likely to be retrieved.

Currently, microdissection TESE is the gold standard for sperm retrieval in men with NOA, against which all future techniques and modifications will have to be compared.

4.4 Future Directions

The history of surgical sperm retrieval is not complete. Though a variety of techniques have been developed, ranging in invasiveness and efficacy, our current techniques are still crude. In the future, we should hope to have methods that could identify which men with NOA have sperm in their testes, and non-invasively pin-point focal areas of sperm production. Various biomarkers are being investigated as promising potential indicators of spermatogenesis in men with NOA [44–48]. Techniques under investigation to localize sperm-bearing tubules include multiphoton microscopy [49], full-field optical coherent tomography [50], and tissue perfusion monitoring using narrowband imaging [51].

Surgical sperm retrieval, especially in men with NOA, continues to be a challenging area and future techniques should result in more precise approaches to finding sperm.

References

1. Esteves SC, Roque M, Garrido N. Use of testicular sperm for intracytoplasmic sperm injection in men with high sperm DNA fragmentation: a SWOT analysis. *Asian J Androl* 2018;20:1–8.

2. Mehta A, Esteves SC, Schlegel PN, et al. Use of testicular sperm in nonazoospermic males. *Fertil Steril* 2018;109:981–987.

3. Hanley HG. The surgery of male subfertility: Hunterian lecture delivered at the Royal College of Surgeons of England on 24th May 1955. *Ann R Coll Surg Engl* 1955;17(3):159–183.

4. Momen MN, Roaiah MF. Alloplastic spermatocele in cases of vasa aplasia. *Arch Androl* 1985;14:89–91.

5. Jimenez Cruz JF. Artificial spermatocele. *J Urol* 1980;123:885–886.

6. Kelâmi A. Kelâmi-Affeld alloplastic spermatocele and successful human delivery. *Urol Int* 1981;36:368–372.

7. Temple-Smith PD, Southwick GJ, Yates CA, Trounson AO, de Kretser DM. Human pregnancy by in vitro fertilization (IVF) using sperm aspirated from the epididymis. *J In Vitro Fert Embryo Transf* 1985;2:119–122.

8. Silber S, Ord T, Borrero C, Balmaceda J, Asch R. New treatment for infertility due to congenital absence of vas deferens. *Lancet* 1987;10(2):850–851

9. Silber SJ, Nagy ZP, Liu J, et al. Conventional in-vitro fertilization versus intracytoplasmic sperm injection for patients requiring microsurgical sperm aspiration. *Hum Reprod* 1994;9:1705–1709.

10. Tsirigotis M, Bennett V, Hogewind G, Pelekanos M, Craft I. Percutaneous epididymal sperm aspiration simplified sperm recovery for obstructive azoospermia. *Hum Reprod* 1994;9:169–170.

11. Shrivastav P, Nadkarni P, Wensvoort S, Craft I. Percutaneous epididymal sperm aspiration for obstructive azoospermia. *Hum Reprod* 1994;9:2058–2061.

12. Craft I, Tsirigotis M, Bennett V, et al. Percutaneous epididymal sperm aspiration and intracytoplasmic sperm injection in the management of infertility due to obstructive azoospermia. *Fertil Steril* 1995;63:1038–1042.

13. Shah RS. Surgical and non-surgical methods of sperm retrieval. In Hansotia M, Desai S, Parihar M (eds.) *Advanced Infertility Management.* Jaypee Brothers, New Delhi, 2002, pp. 253–258.

14. Craft I, Bennett V, Nicholson N. Fertilising ability of testicular spermatozoa. *Lancet* 1993;342 (8875):864

15. Schoysman R, Vanderzwalmen P, Nijs M, et al. Pregnancy after fertilization with human testicular spermatozoa. *Lancet* 1993;342:1237.

16. Devroey P, Liu J, Nagy Z, et al. Normal fertilization of human oocytes after testicular sperm extraction and intracytoplasmic sperm injection. *Fertil Steril* 1994;62:639–641.

17. Nagy Z, Liu J, Cecile J, et al. Using ejaculated, fresh, and frozen–thawed epididymal and testicular spermatozoa gives rise to comparable results after intracytoplasmic sperm injection. *Fertil Steril* 1995;63:808–815.

18. Levin HS. Testicular biopsy in the study of male infertility: its current usefulness, histologic techniques, and prospects for the future. *Hum Pathol* 1979;10:569–584.

19. Devroey P, Liu J, Nagy Z, et al. Pregnancies after testicular sperm extraction and intracytoplasmic sperm injection in non-obstructive azoospermia. *Hum Reprod* 1995;10:1457–1460.

20. Yemini M, Vanderzwalmen P, Mukaida T, Schoengold S, Birkenfeld A. Intracytoplasmic sperm injection, fertilization, and embryo transfer after retrieval of spermatozoa by testicular biopsy from an azoospermic male with testicular tubular atrophy. *Fertil Steril* 1995;63:1118–1120.

21. Gil-Salom M, Remohí J, Mínguez Y, Rubio C, Pellicer A. Pregnancy in an azoospermic patient with markedly elevated serum follicle-stimulating hormone levels. *Fertil Steril* 1995;64:1218–1220.

22. Tournaye H, Liu J, Nagy PZ, et al. Correlation between testicular histology and outcome after intracytoplasmic sperm injection using testicular spermatozoa. *Hum Reprod* 1996;11:127–132.

23. Shah R. 1935: the single seminiferous tubule (SST) technique for atraumatic multiple testicular biopsies for sperm retrieval. *J Urol* 2004;171(4S):511

24. Obrant KO, Persson PS. Cytological study of the testis by aspiration biopsy in the evaluation of fertility. *Urol Int* 1965;20:176–189.

25. Lewin A, Weiss DB, Friedler S, et al. Delivery following intracytoplasmic injection of mature sperm cells recovered by testicular fine needle aspiration in a case of hypergonadotropic azoospermia due to maturation arrest. *Hum Reprod* 1996;11 (4):769–771.

26. Lewin A, Reubinoff B, Porat-Katz A, et al. Testicular fine needle aspiration: the alternative method for sperm retrieval in non-obstructive azoospermia. *Hum Reprod* 1999;14:1785–1790.

27. Friedler S, Raziel A, Strassburger D, et al. Testicular sperm retrieval by percutaneous fine needle sperm aspiration compared with testicular sperm extraction by open biopsy in men with non-obstructive azoospermia. *Hum Reprod* 1997;12:1488–1493.

28. Foresta C, Garolla A, Bettella A, et al. Doppler ultrasound of the testis in azoospermic subjects as a parameter of testicular function. *Hum Reprod* 1998;13:3090–3093.

29. Har-Toov J, Eytan O, Hauser R, et al. A new power Doppler ultrasound guiding technique for improved testicular sperm extraction. *Fertil Steril* 2004;81:430–434.

30. Herwig R, Tosun K, Schuster A, et al. Tissue perfusion-controlled guided biopsies are essential for the outcome of testicular sperm extraction. *Fertil Steril* 2007;87:1071–1076.

23

31. Morey AF, Deshon GE Jr, Rozanski TA, Dresner ML. Technique of biopty gun testis needle biopsy. *Urology* 1993;42:325–326.

32. Mallidis C, Baker HW. Fine needle tissue aspiration biopsy of the testis. *Fertil Steril* 1994;61:367–375.

33. Ezeh UI, Moore HD, Cooke ID. A prospective study of multiple needle biopsies versus a single open biopsy for testicular sperm extraction in men with non-obstructive azoospermia. *Hum Reprod* 1998;13:3075–3080.

34. Schlegel PN, Su L-M Physiologic consequences of testicular sperm extraction. *Hum Reprod* 1997;12:1688–1692.

35. Schlegel PN. Testicular sperm extraction: microdissection improves sperm yield with minimal tissue excision. *Hum Reprod* 1999;14:131–135.

36. Deruyver Y, Vanderschueren D, Aa F. Outcome of microdissection TESE compared with conventional TESE in non-obstructive azoospermia: a systematic review. *Andrology* 2014;2:20–24.

37. Ghalayini IF, Al-Ghazo MA, Hani OB, et al. Clinical comparison of conventional testicular sperm extraction and microdissection techniques for non-obstructive azoospermia. *J Clin Med Res* 2011;3:124–131.

38. Maglia E, Boeri L, Fontana M, et al. Clinical comparison between conventional and microdissection testicular sperm extraction for non-obstructive azoospermia: understanding which treatment works for which patient. *Arch Ital Urol Androl* 2018;90: 130–135.

39. Everaert K, De Croo I, Kerckhaert W, et al. Long term effects of micro-surgical testicular sperm extraction on androgen status in patients with non obstructive azoospermia. *BMC Urol* 2006;6:9.

40. Eliveld J, van Wely M, Meißner A, et al. The risk of TESE-induced hypogonadism: a systematic review and meta-analysis. *Hum Reprod Update* 2018;24:442–454.

41. Shah R. Surgical sperm retrieval: techniques and their indications. *Ind J Urol* 2011;27:102–109.

42. Franco G, Scarselli F, Casciani V, et al. A novel stepwise micro-TESE approach in non obstructive azoospermia. *BMC Urol* 2016;16:20.

43. Shin DH, Turek PJ. Sperm retrieval techniques. *Nat Rev Urol* 2013;10:723–730.

44. Fukuda T, Miyake H, Enatsu N, Matsushita K, Fujisawa M. Seminal level of clusterin in infertile men as a significant biomarker reflecting spermatogenesis. *Andrologia* 2016;48:1188–1194.

45. Alfano M, Ventimiglia E, Locatelli I, et al. Anti-Mullerian hormone-to-testosterone ratio is predictive of positive sperm retrieval in men with idiopathic non-obstructive azoospermia. *Sci Rep* 2017;7:17638.

46. Gilany K, Mani-Varnosfaderani A, Minai-Tehrani A, et al. Untargeted metabolomic profiling of seminal plasma in nonobstructive azoospermia men: a noninvasive detection of spermatogenesis. *Biomed Chromatogr* 2017;31(8). doi: 10.1002/bmc.3931.

47. Cao C, Wen Y, Wang X, et al. Testicular piRNA profile comparison between successful and unsuccessful micro-TESE retrieval in NOA patients. *J Assist Reprod Genet* 2018;35:801–808.

48. Hashemi MS, Mozdarani H, Ghaedi K, Nasr-Esfahani MH. Expression of ZMYND15 in testes of azoospermic men and association with sperm retrieval. *Urology* 2018;114:99–104.

49. Ramasamy R, Sterling J, Fisher ES, et al. Identification of spermatogenesis with multiphoton microscopy: an evaluation in a rodent model. *J Urol* 2011;186:2487–2492.

50. Ramasamy R, Sterling J, Manzoor M, et al. Full field optical coherence tomography can identify spermatogenesis in a rodent Sertoli-cell only model. *J Pathol Inform* 2012;3:4.

51. Enatsu N, Miyake H, Chiba K, Fujisawa M. Identification of spermatogenically active regions in rat testes by using narrow band imaging system. *Urology* 2015;86:929–935.

5

Epididymal Sperm Retrieval
Indications, Surgical Protocol, and Outcomes

Jason P. Akerman and R. Matthew Coward

5.1 Introduction

Azoospermia is diagnosed in approximately 1 percent of the general population and in up to 15 percent of infertile men. Of these men, 15–20 percent can be further categorized as having obstructive azoospermia [1]. Men with obstructive azoospermia have preserved spermatogenesis, allowing for either surgical repair of their obstruction or sperm retrieval to be used in conjunction with *in vitro* fertilization (IVF) with intracytoplasmic sperm injection (ICSI). The obstruction can occur anywhere along the passage of sperm from the efferent ducts within the testis, along the epididymis, through the vas deferens, the ejaculatory ducts, or the distal penile urethra. Causes of obstructive azoospermia can be congenital, acquired, or idiopathic (Table 5.1) [2]. Vasectomy and iatrogenic obstruction to the vas deferens at the time of inguinal hernia repair are the most common causes of acquired obstructive azoospermia. Congenital bilateral absence of the vas deferens (CBAVD) is the most common congenital

cause [3,4]. In men with obstruction of the epididymis or vas deferens, microsurgical reanastomosis at the site of obstruction can be done with good fertility-related outcomes. Those who do not wish to undergo surgical repair of their obstruction, have failed surgical repair, have CBAVD, or have an unclear/multifactorial cause of their obstruction can be treated with sperm retrieval and ICSI [5]. Percutaneous epididymal sperm aspiration (PESA), microsurgical epididymal sperm aspiration (MESA), and the recently described minimally invasive epididymal sperm aspiration (MIESA), are all techniques that allow successful retrieval of sperm from the epididymis in men with obstructive azoospermia (Table 5.2).

5.2 Anatomy of the Epididymis

5.2.1 Structure

Convergence of a series of tubules within the testes, known as the efferent ducts, gives rise to the epididymis [6]. It is located along the posterolateral surface of the testicle and is contained within the visceral tunica vaginalis [7]. The gross appearance of the epididymis is that of a tightly coiled tube that can be divided into the caput, corpus, and cauda. Altogether, it measures 3–4 m in length. Moving from the caput to the cauda, there is a progressive increase in the diameter of the epididymal lumen and thickness of surrounding smooth muscle [7]. This surrounding smooth muscle contracts rhythmically to propel contents forward. Each region of the epididymis is further subdivided by connective-tissue septa that create unique micro-environments and provide structural support [6,8]. As sperm pass through these segments, they experience gains in function and motility [9]. Protection of germ cells from host immunity extends from the testicle to the epididymis in the form of the blood–epididymis barrier. A complex interaction of structural, physiological, and immunological factors

Table 5.1 Common causes of obstructive azoospermia

Acquired	Infectious • Epididymitis, prostatitis Iatrogenic • Vasectomy, previous scrotal surgery, inguinal hernia repair • Vasotomy or vasography (improper technique) Trauma Young syndrome Ejaculatory duct obstruction
Congenital	Congenital unilateral and bilateral absence of vas deferens Absence (partial or complete) of the epididymis Ejaculatory duct cysts
Idiopathic	

Table 5.2 Advantages and disadvantages of approaches to epididymal sperm aspiration

	Advantages	Disadvantages
PESA	No microsurgical skills required Local anesthesia Noninvasive Short operative time Lowest cost	Sperm retrieved in lower quantity and quality compared to MESA Risk of vascular injury due to blind nature of procedure Failure rate of up to 20%
MESA	Microsurgical approach allows higher-quality sperm to be identified Near 100% sperm retrieval rate Sperm can be cryopreserved Higher quantity and more motility compared to PESA sperm Minimal contamination of specimens	General anesthesia Longer operative times compared to PESA Operative microscope and microsurgical skills required Obliterative MESA: obliteration of epididymal retrieval site precludes future reversal or retrieval in that area Longer convalescence compared to PESA
MIESA	Shares the advantages of the MESA approach No microsurgical skills required Local anesthesia with oral sedation Lower cost than conventional MESA	Longer operative times compared to PESA Obliteration of epididymal retrieval site precludes future reversal or retrieval in that area Special training required Often requires monitored anesthesia care

PESA: Percutaneous epididymal sperm aspiration
MESA: microsurgical epididymal sperm aspiration
MIESA: minimally invasive epididymal sperm aspiration

separates the epididymal lumen from the surrounding vasculature [10].

5.2.2 Arterial Supply of the Epididymis

An understanding of blood supply to the testis and epididymis is required to limit complications during scrotal surgery. While there is some variability in the exact vascular pattern supplying the epididymis, a number of consistencies exist at each segment. In a series of 27 adult specimens, Macmillan characterized the arterial pattern of the human epididymis [11]. The report describes a single epididymal arterial branch at both the caput and corpus of the epididymis. These vessels, termed the superior and inferior epididymal branches, arise from the testicular artery. Their origin may be off of the main trunk of the testicular artery or from one of its main divisions high in the inguinal canal. In the region of the caput, it gives off one or more small capital arteries before descending to the cauda.

There are a variable number of branches to the corpus of the epididymis. This results in an arterial network of convoluted and anastomosing arteries. Along the course of the epididymis, branches from the arterial arcade penetrate within the connective-tissue septae with an extensive amount of coiling.

These coiled segments ultimately terminate in a microvascular bed within the epididymis [12]. At the cauda, an anastomotic loop is often observed between the epididymal artery and the vasal artery. The exact distribution and origin of arteries in this region is more variable. Blood supply in the region of the cauda is characterized by communications and anastomoses between the epididymal, vasal, cremasteric, and testicular arteries [11].

5.2.3 Venous Drainage

Veins at the caput of the epididymis drain directly into the pampiniform plexus within the scrotum. A portion of these veins may communicate with the venous drainage of the corpus and cauda of the epididymis. Veins from the remaining portions of the epididymis converge to form the vena marginalis epididymis of Haberer [11].

5.2.4 Lymphatic Drainage

The lymphatic drainage of the epididymis involves a small number of channels arising primarily from the caput. There is a gradual decrease in the number of lymphatics toward the cauda [13]. Channels from the proximal epididymis will merge with those draining the vas deferens and ultimately enter the external iliac nodes. Lymphatics draining the caput and corpus epididymis empty into the pre-aortic nodes [7].

5.3 Indications, Patient Selection, and Uses of Epididymal Sperm

An appropriately selected patient for epididymal sperm aspiration must have either documented or strong clinical suspicion for obstructive azoospermia. Specifically to target epididymal sperm, the patient should have obstruction somewhere between the scrotal vas deferens and the testis (e.g., patients with CBAVD, epididymal obstruction, or vasectomy). Patients with inguinal obstruction and ejaculatory duct obstruction may not have adequate epididymal obstruction and induration to allow for sufficient retrieval from the epididymis and are thus not good candidates for epididymal sperm extraction. The site of obstruction is determined through a thorough male reproductive history, physical examination, and baseline laboratory studies. Determining the most likely site of obstruction also helps determine the etiology, and this crucial information guides the discussion of options. Men with CBAVD may be managed differently from those with a history of vasectomy, for example. In the case of CBAVD, a more thorough exploration with potential conversion to testicular sperm extraction may be required to find adequate sperm, while a man with a prior vasectomy may opt for vasovasostomy.

An azoospermic patient with normal testicular volume, palpable vasa, and a normal follicle-stimulating hormone (FSH) level should have retrograde ejaculation ruled out if semen volume is low or borderline low. In the absence of retrograde ejaculation, transrectal ultrasound should be performed to evaluate for an ejaculatory duct obstruction. If idiopathic or bilateral epididymal obstruction is suspected, even in the absence of a vasal anomaly, mutations of the cystic fibrosis transmembrane conductance regulator gene should be assessed.

Of those men who go on to have some form of epididymal sperm retrieval, there are a few clinical predictors of success. Multivariate analysis of a large sample of men with obstructive azoospermia undergoing PESA found younger age and larger testicular volume to be predictive of motile sperm in the aspirate [14]. While the presence of epididymal cysts in post-vasectomy patients may predict a poor outcome, time since vasectomy and a history of failed

vasovasostomy were not associated with worse epididymal aspirates [15]. The cause of obstructive azoospermia has not been shown to be a reliable predictor of a successful epididymal sperm retrieval [14,15].

5.3.1 Epididymal versus Testicular Sperm for IVF/ICSI

In men with obstructive azoospermia, there is no consensus with respect to the superiority of sperm retrieved from the epididymis or testis for use in IVF/ICSI. Despite promising results of early studies of epididymal sperm, systematic reviews and meta-analyses have failed to find sufficient evidence to recommend one sperm retrieval technique over another [16,17]. Some more recent studies have again suggested a benefit to epididymal-derived sperm. This includes higher live birth rates, pregnancy rates, and implantation rates [18,19]. Epididymal sperm has also been shown to produce more clinically stable blastocysts compared to testicular sperm [19].

There is a growing body of evidence suggesting that levels of DNA fragmentation may be lower in testicular sperm. Among men with high levels of DNA fragmentation in ejaculated samples, testicular sperm may produce better outcomes with ICSI [20]. A small series of men with obstructive azoospermia found similar results. The study noted that DNA fragmentation rates were nearly twice as high in epididymal spermatozoa independent of the cause of obstructive azoospermia [21]. The impact this finding on ICSI outcomes is unclear.

5.3.2 Laboratory Handling of Epididymal Sperm

Sperm retrieved from the epididymis or testis is at high risk of compromise compared to ejaculated samples. Proper handling and sperm processing techniques are required by an experienced lab to maximize the fertility potential of the specimen. Epididymal sperm can be used as either a fresh or frozen–thawed specimen for IVF/ICSI [22]. Processing of epididymal sperm should aim to select the best spermatozoa while optimizing their ability to fertilize. To achieve this, the surgeon must first retrieve a high-quality specimen with minimal contaminants such as red blood cells and microorganisms. The laboratory then needs to apply technical skills to optimize the sperm's environment, including ultraviolet exposure, temperature, laboratory air quality conditions, reagents, culture media, and washing steps [23].

Once obtained, epididymal aspirates are diluted with sperm wash media. This process avoids agglutination of the epididymal spermatozoa and will allow for examination of motile sperm under the microscope. Aspirates should be identified and labeled, including the site of aspiration and the presence or absence of motile sperm. Epididymal sperm may be used for a fresh transfer with ICSI or cryopreserved using similar protocols to those used for ejaculated specimens [22–27]. The cryopreserved epididymal sperm is then resuspended in a small aliquot of medium to allow for identification of motile or twitching sperm. These will then be isolated for use in the ICSI procedure [23,26].

5.3.3 Fresh versus Frozen–Thawed Epididymal Sperm

Use of cryopreserved epididymal sperm to achieve pregnancy was first reported in 1995 as part of a small series comparing frozen and fresh samples [28]. Over the course of the following decades, the use of cryopreserved epididymal sperm has increased significantly. Epididymal sperm retrieved from men with obstructive azoospermia often provide abundant sperm that can then be cryopreserved for future ICSI cycles. Cryopreservation of sperm avoids logistical constraints that can be a barrier to coordination of sperm retrieval with IVF cycles. It also results in a reduction in the number of surgical sperm retrievals per patient [29–31]. This led investigators to test whether cryopreserved epididymal sperm could provide similar outcomes to fresh samples. Rates of fertilization and clinical pregnancy were noted to be similar when compared to fresh samples [27,32–34]. Embryo quality has also been shown to be maintained with cryopreserved epididymal sperm [31,35].

There is, however, a documented effect of cryopreservation on some sperm characteristics, including a reduction in concentration and a decrease in motile counts [35]. Rarely, viable sperm will not be found at the time of thawing, necessitating a fresh retrieval. It is therefore recommended to include a test thaw of cryopreserved epididymal sperm [27]. Fertilization failure using previously cryopreserved epididymal sperm is associated with samples demonstrating poor postthaw motility [36].

5.4 Methods of Epididymal Sperm Aspiration

5.4.1 Percutaneous Epididymal Sperm Aspiration

5.4.1.1 Historical Development and Current Indications

The first use of aspirated epididymal sperm was reported in a 1985 paper by Temple-Smith et al. In it, they describe the case of a 42-year-old man with a history of vasectomy and two subsequent failed reversals with vasoepididymostomy. The patient was ultimately taken back to the operating room a third time for planned fresh transfer in an IVF cycle. Following 90 min of massage at the site of the right ductus epididymis, a total of 0.2 ml was aspirated and found to contain 76 percent motile sperm. Successful fertilization and clinical pregnancy was achieved through IVF [37]. Nearly 10 years later, Craft and Shrivastav described their approach, now known as PESA, in a letter to the editor of the *Lancet*. At the time, few centers had access to the microsurgical equipment required for MESA. The approach obviated the need for surgical microscope, but was still performed with intravenous or general anesthesia [38]. PESA is now commonly performed in the outpatient setting with local anesthesia.

5.4.1.2 Success Rates and Evidence in Support

The success of PESA is highly dependent on the surgeon's ability to correctly identify and diagnose obstructive azoospermia in addition to his or her surgical skill and experience. This includes a history, physical examination, and endocrine profile, as previously outlined. Rates of successful sperm retrieval in men with obstructive azoospermia range from 78 to 100 percent with PESA, irrespective of the cause of their obstruction [39]. Those without a successful PESA will need a second procedure such as a testicular sperm aspiration or extraction. In one of the only comparative studies with PESA as an intervention, Collins et al. performed MESA and PESA on both testes in men with previously proven fertility seeking vasectomy reversal. There was no difference in the rate of successful sperm retrieval between MESA and PESA. Due to its less invasive nature, the authors recommended PESA when possible in this carefully selected group of men with obstructive azoospermia secondary to vasectomy [40].

5.4.1.3 Anesthetic Selection

PESA is performed with local anesthesia, with or without oral sedation. Oral sedation may consist of a combination of an anxiolytic and narcotic medication. With this combination of sedation and anesthesia, it is critical that surgeons and their support staff acquire training in office-based sedation safety. Appropriate monitoring and reversal agents should be readily available.

In keeping with current best practices as outlined in the American Urological Association's guideline "Urologic Procedures and Antimicrobial Prophylaxis," a single dose of cephalosporin is administered to patients. Ampicillin/sulbactam may be considered in those who are unable to tolerate a first-generation cephalosporin.

5.4.1.4 Procedure

Anesthetic Agents

Local anesthesia at the time of surgery is achieved through a combination of a spermatic cord block, superficial pudendal block, and peri-incisional infiltration of anesthetic. The anesthetic itself is often chosen by surgeon preference. Lidocaine and bupivacaine are commonly used anesthetics in scrotal surgery due to their favorable pharmacodynamics and pharmacokinetics. A combination of lidocaine and bupivacaine (1 percent lidocaine in a 1:1 ratio with 0.25 percent bupivacaine, both without epinephrine) provides excellent anesthesia for office-based sperm aspiration. This provides a local anesthetic with an onset of less than 30 s and a duration of approximately 7 h. Maximum doses are 4 mg/kg of lidocaine without epinephrine and 2 mg/kg of bupivacaine without epinephrine. The typical epididymal sperm retrieval procedure requires approximately 10–20 ml of this anesthetic combination.

Spermatic Cord Block, Superficial Pudendal Block

The procedure begins with a well-performed spermatic cord block. This technique was described by Wakefield and Elewa [41]. With the non-dominant hand, the vas deferens is isolated between the thumb and index finger while elevating the entire cord. The vas deferens is maintained posteriorly while the spermatic cord is held tightly against the scrotal skin in an anterior fashion. Local anesthetic is infiltrated with a 25-gauge, 1.5-inch needle attached to a 10 ml syringe, which has been pre-filled with a 1:1 mixture of 1 percent lidocaine and 0.25 percent bupivacaine (both without epinephrine). The needle is inserted at a point 1 cm below and medial to the pubic tubercle in the direction of the high spermatic cord. As the needle is advanced toward and then into the cord, the anesthetic is continuously and slowly injected. In doing so, the anesthetic creates a hydro-dissecting effect that clears vessels along its course. Approximately three passes of the needle are made into the cord in a fan-like distribution. Superficial branches of the pudendal nerve are then blocked using the remaining local anesthetic. This is done by subcutaneous infiltration lateral to the cord along the scrotal–inguinal plane. The combination of a spermatic cord block and superficial pudendal block typically requires 10 ml of the anesthetic mixture. Finally, a peri-incisional block along the planned skin incision is done using the same syringe, needle, and solution.

Procedure

Sperm aspiration is done using a 21- or 23-gauge butterfly needle. The needle is first connected to a 20 ml syringe and primed with 1 ml of sperm wash medium. Before the epididymis is infiltrated with the needle, negative pressure suction is obtained within the system. The needle is passed into the upper scrotum at the anesthetized skin site, and then maximum suction is applied to the syringe (Figure 5.1). A hemostat is placed across the tubing of the butterfly needle in order to maintain suction. With the butterfly needle in the scrotum, the caput of the epididymis is repositioned. This is done by positioning the epididymis between the thumb and finger and orienting it toward the needle. Once appropriately positioned in the epididymis, the hemostat is released. This allows the vacuum within the needle system to draw sperm into the tubing. The needle is repositioned multiple times without withdrawing it from the scrotum. This is critical to maintaining negative pressure in the system and to allowing the maximum amount of sperm to be collected in the aspirate. The needle is then removed and direct pressure is applied to the site of entry.

An aliquot of the sperm aspirate is examined on a slide by the embryologist for motile sperm. If needed, the procedure may be repeated on the contralateral side. The amount of viable sperm retrieved may not be sufficient for cryopreservation and will go on to be used immediately for ICSI.

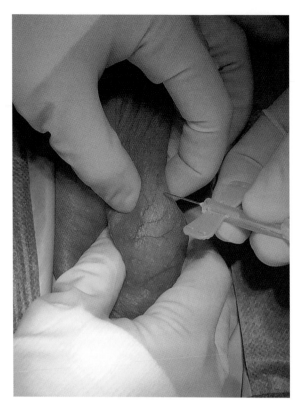

Figure 5.1 Percutaneous needle insertion during a PESA procedure.

5.4.1.5 Advantages, Disadvantages, Complications

The percutaneous nature of this procedure is appealing and allows it to be performed on short notice under local anesthesia. A short recovery time for patients, perceived ease of successfully retrieving sperm, and its reproducibility are other factors that make this form of sperm retrieval attractive to both surgeons and patients. Unlike other methods of sperm retrieval, PESA does not require special equipment or training in microsurgery.

The procedure does, however, come with a number of disadvantages. If we assume a failure rate of 20 percent, as has been observed in the published literature, a significant number of patients will require an additional and more invasive surgical sperm retrieval. A failed PESA can have significant consequences for coordination with an IVF cycle, operating room scheduling, and added patient burden. Aspirates from PESA have fewer sperm with an average motility lower than what is seen with open, direct epididymal sperm extraction techniques described later [42].

Overall common complication rates with PESA are low and include pain, hydrocele, infection, and swelling. Epididymal obstruction and theoretical damage to the testicular artery at its insertion site beneath the caput of the epididymis are other potential complications [42]. Due to its blind nature, there is a higher risk of vascular injury at the time of PESA compared to other methods of sperm retrieval [42].

5.4.2 Microsurgical Epididymal Sperm Aspiration

5.4.2.1 Historical Development and Current Indications

Microsurgical aspiration of epididymal sperm was first described in a 1988 paper by Silber et al. In it, they outline a technique for epididymal sperm aspiration under 10–40× magnification that begins in the distal corpus of the epididymis and continues proximally until motile sperm are retrieved. The two patients in which this procedure was initially described both had CBAVD [43]. This new technique, to be used in conjunction with IVF, was well received and offered a path to pregnancy for men with obstructive azoospermia. Early fertilization and pregnancy rates, however, did not produce favorable results, with many centers reporting a success rate under 10 percent. The advent of ICSI a few years later led to significant improvements in outcomes with epididymal sperm [44]. With these changes came renewed interest in the MESA technique. MESA has since become the gold standard approach for sperm retrieval in men with obstructive azoospermia.

5.4.2.2 Success Rates and Evidence in Support

Microsurgical epididymal sperm aspiration is well supported as a method of epididymal sperm retrieval that provides large quantities of high-quality sperm. Retrieval rates in appropriately selected men with obstructive azoospermia approach 100 percent. The number of sperm retrieved far exceeds those required for a single ICSI/IVF cycle, and they can be cryopreserved in 98–100 percent of cases. On average, MESA yields 15–95 million total sperm, with 15–42 percent total motility [45,46]. Combined with ICSI, epididymal sperm obtained by MESA has a clinical pregnancy rate of 42–60 percent [46,47].

5.4.2.3 Procedure
Anesthetic Selection

Several techniques for MESA have been reported, including some in an outpatient office-based setting.

A conventional MESA is performed under general anesthesia in an operating room.

Surgical Approach

The technique of a conventional MESA, as described by Goldstein, can be used for intraoperative sperm at the time of vasoepididymostomy or in appropriately selected men with obstructive azoospermia [5]. A high transverse hemiscrotal incision, vertical paramedian incision, or midline scrotal incision may be utilized. The larger or heathier appearing testis is typically selected for the procedure. A bilateral approach is rarely required or indicated.

Following dissection through the dartos layer, the tunica vaginalis is opened sharply to allow for evaluation of the epididymis under an operating microscope. This is typically done under a magnification of 16–25×, based on surgeon preference. The magnified epididymis is inspected for dilated tubules. Those containing white or clear fluid are more likely to contain motile sperm and are selected for aspiration [42]. Once identified, the epididymal tunic overlying the desired tubules is incised. This is done with a 15-degree ophthalmic microknife. In men with a history of prior vasectomy, a secondary obstruction or "blow-out" may be identified. This presents as a transition change in the appearance and size of the tubules. A location proximal to this secondary obstruction is more likely to be successful in identifying motile sperm.

The aspirated fluid from the incised tubule is then placed onto a slide with sperm wash media. If no motile sperm are seen on the slide, both the tunica and epididymal tubule are closed. Subsequent incisions are made, moving proximally on the epididymis. In cases of prolonged obstruction, the highest-quality sperm is generally found in the caput of the epididymis. For example, the best sperm for aspiration are found near the efferent ducts in men with CBAVD. Once motile sperm are confirmed, micropipettes are used to aspirate from the site of the open tubule. Gentle massage of the epididymis may help to express additional fluid to be aspirated. Closure of the tunica vaginalis is done in running fashion with an absorbable 3-0 or 4-0 suture before returning the testicle to within the scrotum.

"Obliterative" MESA

In response to concerns that selective aspiration with micropipette may limit the sperm yield of a conventional MESA, Larry Lipshultz developed and popularized a modified technique. Eventually coined the "obliterative MESA" by Karpman et al., this approach sought to maximize collection in order to allow for cryopreservation of larger numbers of high-quality sperm [48].

The procedure begins the same way as a conventional MESA up until the epididymal tubules are exposed. Incision of the desired tubules is carried out as described above. Once motile sperm are found, the maximum number of tubules proximal to this point are incised. This exhausts all potential sites for sperm retrieval, leading to larger yields than a conventional MESA. It is therefore important that patients understand that an obliterative MESA renders further epididymal retrieval or reconstruction impossible.

With the tubule incised, an assistant uses a tuberculin syringe with a 24-gauge angiocatheter tip primed with sperm wash media to aspirate the fluid. Instead of closing the incision sites, electrocautery is used to obtain hemostasis and effectively obliterate the retrieval sites. This is accomplished by sweeping the cautery over the epididymal tissue in a manner similar to that used in renal sparing surgeries. After hemostasis is assured, the tunica vaginalis is closed with 3-0 chromic and the testicle is returned to the scrotum. Dartos fascia and skin are each closed with 3-0 chromic in a running fashion.

5.4.2.4 Advantages, Disadvantages, Complications

Microsurgical epididymal sperm aspiration is widely considered the gold standard for sperm retrieval in men with obstructive azoospermia. The primary advantages of this approach are its near-uniform acquisition of large numbers of high-quality sperm, ability to cryopreserve sperm for future use, minimal contamination of sperm, quick recovery, and low rate of complications. Other than pain, bleeding and infection are the most common complications. These occur at a rate of <1 percent [45,49]. Unlike PESA, MESA allows for a more thorough evaluation of epididymal tubules and selection of those with the best quality sperm.

Despite its advantages, MESA should not be seen as the only solution for all men with obstructive azoospermia. Men with a history of vasectomy, for example, may have other appropriate options for their infertility. Vasovasostomy remains a gold standard surgical solution for these men, even in the era of ICSI. It has been found to produce more favorable pregnancy rates in cost–benefit analyses and removes the morbidity of an IVF/ICSI cycle for the female partner [50]. In this post-vasectomy population, PESA produced similar rates of sperm retrieval through a less invasive approach and should also be considered [40].

The disadvantages of MESA are primarily related to the equipment and expertise required, as well as its more invasive nature. As the conventional approach necessitates an open surgical procedure under general anesthesia, there is an associated increased morbidity. Scheduling a MESA with oocyte retrieval can be a challenge for the urologist and requires more operative time than a percutaneous approach. It also requires additional training in microsurgery.

5.4.3 Minimally Invasive Epididymal Sperm Aspiration

5.4.3.1 Historical Development

Since the introduction of MESA, attempts have been made to reduce the morbidity and costs associated with this form of sperm retrieval. Examples include the "mini-micro-epididymal sperm aspiration" and the "mini-MESA"[29,48]. While both of these techniques used smaller incisions to reduce morbidity, the procedure required the use of an operating microscope and general anesthesia. The MIESA, as described by Coward and Mills, further simplifies epididymal sperm retrieval without compromising sperm yields. Depending on surgeon preference, MIESA can be pronounced the same as "MESA," or with a distinct pronunciation like "Me-ay-sa" [39].

5.4.3.2 Benefits of this Emerging Technique

The MIESA technique further reduces patient morbidity by utilizing a 1 cm keyhole incision that adequately exposes the epididymis without delivering the testicle. It does not require the use of general anesthesia or an operating microscope, allowing it to be performed in the office setting. This can produce significant cost savings when compared to a conventional MESA under general anesthesia.

5.4.3.3 Anesthesia

In the office setting, oral sedation or monitored anesthesia care (MAC) is administered. This is used in conjunction with local anesthesia. Typically, a spermatic cord block with superficial pudendal nerve block and peri-incisional skin block is performed at the beginning of the case. A description of this technique is outlined earlier in this chapter. The combination of local and oral sedation provides sufficient patient comfort throughout the procedure and allows it to be performed in the office setting without general anesthesia.

5.4.3.4 Procedure and Surgical Approach

Although no operating microscope is required, magnification with surgical loupes is recommended. A 1 cm transverse upper hemiscrotal incision is made down through the dartos layer. It is critical that during the incision an assistant orients the testis to allow entry at the superior aspect of the tunica vaginalis. This will facilitate easy identification and exposure of the epididymis. When the tunica vaginalis is reached, entry is performed sharply. Placing hemostats on either side of the vaginalis at the site of entry will help with appropriate orientation for closure at the end of the case.

The caput of the epididymis is then exposed and delivered. Occasionally, a stay suture is placed in the upper third of the corpus. Additional local anesthetic to the peripheral epididymal tunic may be required at this time for those patients not under MAC. An eyelid retractor may be positioned to maximize exposure. Exposure and positioning are demonstrated in Figure 5.2. Selection of the appropriate location for epididymotomy is done in a similar fashion to that described in the section on conventional MESA. The authors prefer a version of the obliterative MESA technique of aspiration to maximize the amount of sperm retrieved.

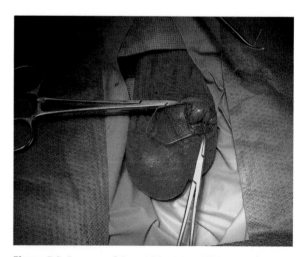

Figure 5.2 Exposure of the epididymis in a MIESA procedure.

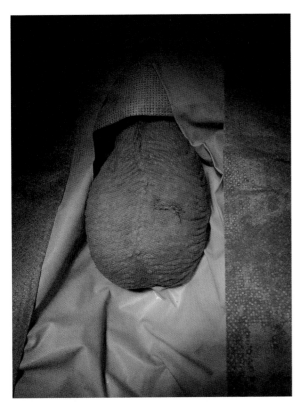

Figure 5.3 Closure of skin in MIESA procedure.

A 15-degree double-beveled ophthalmic knife is passed directly through the epididymal tunic and into a predetermined tubule with a slow, steady motion. Fluid from the initial puncture is placed on a slide for evaluation by the embryologist. Incisions proceed proximally until motile sperm are observed. An obliterative MESA-like approach is then used to target all tubules more proximal to this site.

Hemostasis is obtained with electrocautery over each epididymotomy site. As outlined in the section on obliterative MESA, sweeping electrocautery is then used to obliterate the opened portion of the epididymis. As the tunica vaginalis is closed, additional local anesthetic is injected to create a small hydrocele-like collection around the testis. Closure of both the dartos fascia and skin is done in a running fashion with 3-0 chromic sutures (Figure 5.3).

5.5 Conclusions

For men with obstructive azoospermia pursuing IVF/ICSI with surgically extracted sperm, epididymal sperm provides excellent outcomes equal if not superior to sperm retrieved from the testis. Men with obstructive azoospermia have a number of options for epididymal sperm retrieval that are reliable and reproducible in the hands of fellowship-trained male fertility specialists. In addition to a discussion of the benefits and shortcomings of the various procedures, patients should be made aware of appropriate alternatives to sperm retrieval with IVF/ICSI. This would include, for example, a discussion of vasovasostomy in men with a history of vasectomy. While PESA is the cheapest and least invasive, it may be best suited to fresh transfers with IVF/ICSI or when sperm is required on short notice. Both MESA and MIESA offer excellent retrieval rates of high-quality sperm that can be used both in a fresh IVF cycle and cryopreserved for future cycles. MIESA is a particularly promising retrieval technique as it reduces the morbidity of a conventional MESA without compromising the quality and quantity of sperm obtained.

References

1. Jarow JP, Espeland MA, Lipshultz LI. Evaluation of the azoospermic patient. *J Urol* 1989;142(1): 62–65.

2. Wosnitzer MS, Goldstein M. Obstructive azoospermia. *Urol Clin North Am* 2014;41(1): 83–95.

3. Sheynkin YR, Hendin BN, Schlegel PN, Goldstein M. Microsurgical repair of iatrogenic injury to the vas deferens. *J Urol* 1998;159:139–141.

4. Hussein TM, Zakaria NH, Zahran AM. Clinical, laboratory and genetic assessment of patients with congenital bilateral absent vas deferens. *Andrologia* 2011. doi:10.1111/j.1439-0272.2009.01001.x.

5. Goldstein M. Surgical management of male infertility. *Campbell-Walsh Urology*, 11th edn., Elsevier, Amsterdam, 2012, pp. 648–687.

6. Robaire B, Hinton BT. The epididymis. In: *Knobil and Neill's Physiology of Reproduction.* Academic Press, New York, 2014, pp. 691–771.

7. Kavoussi PK. Surgical, radiographic and endoscopic anatomy of the male reproductive system *Campbell–Walsh Urology*, 11th edn., Elsevier, Amsterdam, 2012, pp. 498–515.e2.

8. Turner TT, Johnston DS, Jelinsky SA, Tomsig JL, Finger JN. Segment boundaries of the adult rat epididymis limit interstitial

signaling by potential paracrine factors and segments lose differential gene expression after efferent duct ligation. *Asian J Androl* 2007;9:565–573.

9. Robaire B, Hamzeh M. Androgen action in the epididymis. *J Androl* 2011;32:592–599.

10. Agarwal A, Hoffer AP. Ultrastructural studies on the development of the blood–epididymis barrier in immature rats. *J Androl* 1989;10:425–431.

11. Macmillan EW. The blood supply of the epididymis in man. *Br J Urol* 1954;26:60–71.

12. Kormano M, Reijonen K. Microvascular structure of the human epididymis. *Am J Anat* 1976;145:23–27.

13. Parez-Clavier R, Harrison RG, Macmillan EW. The pattern of the lymphatic drainage of the rat epididymis. *J Anat* 1982;134:667–675.

14. Yafi FA, Zini A. Percutaneous epididymal sperm aspiration for men with obstructive azoospermia: predictors of successful sperm retrieval. *Urology* 2013;82:341–344.

15. Wood S, Vang E, Troup S, Kingsland CR, Lewis-Jones DI. Surgical sperm retrieval after previous vasectomy and failed reversal: clinical implications for in vitro fertilization. *BJU Int* 2002;90:227–281.

16. Palermo GD, Schlegel PN, Hariprashad JJ, et al. Fertilization and pregnancy outcome with intracytoplasmic sperm injection for azoospermic men. *Hum Reprod* 1999;14:741–748.

17. Nicopoullos JDM, Gilling-Smith C, Almeida PA, et al. Use of surgical sperm retrieval in azoospermic men: a meta-analysis. *Fertil Steril* 2004;82:691–701.

18. van Wely M, Barbey N, Meissner A, Repping S, Silber SJ. Live birth rates after MESA or TESE in men with obstructive azoospermia: is there a difference? *Hum Reprod* 2015;30:761–766.

19. Morin SJ, Hanson BM, Juneau CR, et al. A comparison of the relative efficiency of ICSI and extended culture with epididymal sperm versus testicular sperm in patients with obstructive azoospermia. *Asian J Androl* 2020;22:222–226.

20. Esteves SC, Lee W, Benjamin DJ, et al. Reproductive potential of men with obstructive azoospermia undergoing percutaneous sperm retrieval and intracytoplasmic sperm injection according to the cause of obstruction. *J Urol* 2013;189:232–237.

21. Hammoud I, Bailly M, Bergere M, et al. Testicular spermatozoa are of better quality than epididymal spermatozoa in patients with obstructive azoospermia. *Urology* 2017;103:106–111.

22. Esteves S, Varghese A. Laboratory handling of epididymal and testicular spermatozoa: what can be done to improve sperm injections outcome. *J Hum Reprod Sci* 2012;5:233–243.

23. Gangrade BK. Cryopreservation of testicular and epididymal sperm: techniques and clinical outcomes of assisted conception. *Clinics (Sao Paulo)* 2013;68(Suppl. 1):131–140.

24. Patrizio P. Cryopreservation of epididymal sperm. *Mol Cell Endocrinol* 2000;169:11–14.

25. Justice T, Christensen G. Sperm cryopreservation methods. *Methods Mol Biol* 2013;927:209–215.

26. Anger JT, Gilbert BR, Goldstein M. Cryopreservation of sperm: indications, methods and results. *J Urol* 2003;170:1079–1084.

27. Janzen N, Goldstein M, Schlegel PN, Palermo GD, Rosenwaks Z. Use of electively cryopreserved microsurgically aspirated epididymal sperm with IVF and intracytoplasmic sperm injection for obstructive azoospermia. *Fertil Steril* 2000;74:696–701.

28. Devroey P, Silber S, Nagy Z, et al. Ongoing pregnancies and birth after intracytoplasmic sperm injection with frozen–thawed epididymal spermatozoa. *Hum Reprod* 1995;10:903–906.

29. Nudell DM, Conaghan J, Pedersen RA, et al. The mini-micro-epididymal sperm aspiration for sperm retrieval: a study of urological outcomes. *Hum Reprod* 1998;13:1260–1265.

30. Oates RD, Lobel SM, Harris DH, et al. Efficacy of intracytoplasmic sperm injection using intentionally cryopreserved epididymal spermatozoa. *Hum Reprod* 1996;11:133–138.

31. Wood S, Thomas K, Schnauffer K, et al. Reproductive potential of fresh and cryopreserved epididymal and testicular spermatozoa in consecutive intracytoplasmic sperm injection cycles in the same patients. *Fertil Steril* 2002;77:1162–1166.

32. Friedler S, Raziel A, Soffer Y, et al. The outcome of intracytoplasmic injection of fresh and cryopreserved epididymal spermatozoa from patients with obstructive azoospermia: a comparative study. *Hum Reprod* 1998;13:1872–1877.

33. Hutchon S, Thornton S, Hall J, Bishop M. Frozen–thawed epididymal sperm is effective for intracytoplasmic sperm injection: implications for the urologist. *Br J Urol* 1998;81:607–611.

34. Madgar I, Hourvitz A, Levron J, et al. Outcome of in vitro fertilization and intracytoplasmic injection of epididymal and testicular sperm extracted from patients with obstructive and nonobstructive azoospermia. *Fertil Steril* 1998;69:1080–1084.

35. Cayan S, Lee D, Conaghan J, et al. A comparison of ICSI outcomes with fresh and cryopreserved epididymal spermatozoa from the same couples. *Hum Reprod* 2001;16:495–499.

36. Moomjy M, Scott Sills E, Rosenwaks Z, Palermo GD. Implications of complete fertilization failure after intracytoplasmic sperm injection for subsequent fertilization and reproductive outcome. *Hum Reprod* 1998;13:2212–2216.

37. Temple-Smith PD, Southwick GJ, Yates CA, Trounson AO, de Kretser DM. Human pregnancy by in vitro fertilization (IVF) using sperm aspirated from the epididymis. *J Vitr Fertil Embryo Transf* 1985;2:119–122.

38. Craft I, Shrivastav P, Quinton R, et al. Treatment of male infertility. *Lancet* 1994;344:191–192.

39. Coward RM, Mills JN. A step-by-step guide to office-based sperm retrieval for obstructive azoospermia. *Transl Androl Urol* 2017;6:730–744.

40. Collins GN, Critchlow JD, Lau MW, Payne SR. Open versus closed epididymal sperm retrieval in men with secondarily obstructed vasal systems: a preliminary report. *Br J Urol* 1996;78:437–439.

41. Wakefield SE, Elewa AA. Spermatic cord block: a safe technique for intrascrotal surgery. *Ann R Coll Surg Engl* 1994;76:401–402.

42. Chiles KA, Schlegel PN. Sperm retrieval. In Smith JAJ, Howards SS, Preminger GM, Dmochowski RR (eds.) *Hinman's Atlas of Urologic Surgery*, 4th edn., Elsevier, Amsterdam, 2018, pp. 791–793.

43. Silber SJ, Balmaceda J, Borrero C, Ord T, Asch R. Pregnancy with sperm aspiration from the proximal head of the epididymis: a new treatment for congenital absence of the vas deferens. *Fertil Steril* 1988;50:525–528.

44. Silber SJ, Nagy Z, Liu J, et al. The use of epididymal and testicular spermatozoa for intracytoplasmic sperm injection: the genetic implications for male infertility. *Hum Reprod* 1995;10:2031–2043.

45. Bernie AM, Ramasamy R, Stember DS, Stahl PJ. Microsurgical epididymal sperm aspiration: indications, techniques and outcomes. *Asian J Androl* 2013;15:40–43.

46. Hibi H, Sumitomo M, Fukunaga N, Sonohara M, Asada Y. Superior clinical pregnancy rates after microsurgical epididymal sperm aspiration. *Reprod Med Biol* 2018;17:59–63.

47. Bromage SJ, Falconer DA, Lieberman BA, Sangar V, Payne SR. Sperm retrieval rates in subgroups of primary azoospermic males. *Eur Urol* 2007;51:534–539.

48. Karpman E, Williams D. Techniques of sperm retrieval. In Lipshultz LI, Howard SS, Niederberger CS (eds.) *Infertility in the Male*, 4th edn., Cambridge University Press, New York, 2009. pp. 407–420.

49. Shin DH, Turek PJ. Sperm retrieval techniques. *Nat Rev Urol* 2013;10:723–730.

50. Heidenreich A, Altmann P, Engelmann UH. Microsurgical vasovasostomy versus microsurgical epididymal sperm aspiration/testicular extraction of sperm combined with intracytoplasmic sperm injection: a cost–benefit analysis. *Eur Urol* 2000;37:609–614.

Testicular Sperm Retrieval
Indications, Surgical Protocol, and Outcomes

Ahmad Majzoub, Chak Lam Cho, and Sandro C. Esteves

6.1 Introduction

Surgical sperm retrieval can be considered the single most important breakthrough that the field of male infertility has witnessed. The advancements in assisted reproductive technology (ART) in the 1970s allowed physicians to investigate alternative sources of sperm from men with azoospermia. This clinical condition, defined as the absence of sperm in the ejaculate, is prevalent in about 1 percent of all men and in up to 15 percent of men seeking conception [1]. Nonobstructive azoospermia (NOA) is perhaps the most severe form of male infertility; in the past, men with this condition were considered sterile and adoption or assisted reproduction using donated sperm were the only available options for the couple to become parents. However, in recent years and with the introduction of sperm retrieval techniques, conception was made possible using sperm extracted from the testes of men with NOA. This realization came into action in 1994 after the work of Devroey et al. [2], who retrieved sperm via conventional testicular sperm extraction (cTESE), reporting three pregnancies with intracytoplasmic sperm injection (ICSI). In 1995, Craft and Tsirigotis [3] proposed testicular sperm aspiration (TESA) as a simplified method of sperm recovery for men with NOA. In 1998, and following the reports of a few studies demonstrating the detrimental effects of multiple cTESEs on testicular function [4,5], Schlegel and Li [6] introduced the microsurgical testicular sperm extraction (micro-TESE) method, which allowed the performance of magnified selective biopsies of promising seminiferous tubules, thereby minimizing testicular damage. Finally, in 2001, Shah [7] introduced the single seminiferous tubule (SST) biopsy as a less traumatic alternative method allowing multiple biopsies through puncture holes in the tunica albuginea. This chapter is aimed at describing the indications of testicular sperm retrieval, the surgical techniques, and their clinical outcomes.

6.2 Indications for Testicular Sperm Retrieval

Testicular sperm retrieval can be performed on patients with obstructive azoospermia when attempts at re-canalizing the reproductive tract have failed or are not possible (Table 6.1) [8]. While the retrieval of sperm from the epididymis is favored in such cases, it may fail especially when intratesticular obstruction is present. On the other hand, testicular sperm retrieval is commonly performed for men with NOA in search of focal areas of spermatogenesis. In about 30–60 percent of cases, such areas can be identified, resulting in successful sperm retrieval [9]. Throughout the years, the indications of testicular sperm retrieval have extended to cover conditions other than azoospermia. These include (1) the presence of abnormally high levels of sperm DNA fragmentation; and (2) cryptozoospermia, which is the presence of very few sperm (often with poor quality) in the ejaculate. Sperm DNA fragmentation has been investigated in recent years and the reports have indicated that it plays a crucial role in fertilization, early embryo development, and pregnancy rate [10–14]. It is now believed that high levels of sperm DNA fragmentation could alter the outcome of ART by raising the failure and miscarriage rates following these procedures [15,16]. While sperm DNA fragmentation can occur secondary to defects in chromatin compaction during spermiogenesis, the majority of cases are believed to arise from oxidative stress-related insults during

Table 6.1 Indications of testicular sperm retrieval

Nonobstructive azoospermia

Obstructive azoospermia

High sperm DNA fragmentation

Cryptozoospermia

sperm passage through the male reproductive tract [17–21]. This finding has been confirmed by several studies reporting higher levels of sperm DNA fragmentation in the ejaculates of non-azoospermic men, compared with their intratesticular sperm samples [22–24]. A systemic review by Esteves et al. reported a mean difference in sperm DNA fragmentation rate of –24.6 percent between ejaculate and intratesticular sperm samples [25]. A number of studies have compared the outcome of ICSI using testicular sperm versus ejaculated sperm [22,26,27]. Chapter 8 covers the summary evidence, indications, and protocol concerning testicular sperm retrieval for non-azoospermic men.

Patients with cryptozoospermia ejaculate very few sperm of low motility that may reduce the success rate of ICSI [28]. Therefore, a number of studies have investigated whether testicular sperm retrieval in cases of cryptozoospermia may be associated with improvements in ICSI outcome [28–30]. A recent meta-analysis investigated 761 ICSI cycles performed on men with cryptozoospermia: 541 ICSI cycles with ejaculated sperm, 153 ICSI cycles with fresh testicular sperm, and 67 ICSI cycles with frozen–thawed testicular sperm. The results revealed that testicular sperm did not significantly improve the fertilization rate in comparison to ejaculated sperm (relative risk = 1.08 with 95 percent confidence interval (CI) 0.98–1.32; $p = 0.12$); however, a significant improvement in good-quality embryo rate (1.17, 95 percent CI 1.05–1.30, $p = 0.005$), implantation rate (95 percent CI 1.02–2.26, $p = 0.04$), and pregnancy rate (1.74, 95 percent CI 1.20–2.52, $p = 0.004$) were observed with testicular sperm in comparison to ejaculated sperm in patients with cryptozoospermia [30].

6.3 Surgical Sperm Retrieval

6.3.1 Preoperative Care

Patients should be fully informed about the intended surgical procedure, its potential complications, and the expected outcome before signing the informed surgical consent. Their medical history should be reviewed and optimized before undergoing surgery, especially for patients with diabetes mellitus, cardiac conditions, or bleeding disorders. Antiplatelets, anticoagulants, and nonsteroidal anti-inflammatory medications should preferably be stopped one week before the procedure. Shaving of the scrotal wall hair

should be advised, especially when open surgery is intended. Prophylactic antibiotics (e.g., first-generation cephalosporin) are required, particularly for open procedures.

6.3.2 Anesthesia

Testicular sperm retrieval is a relatively simple procedure that is performed in the operating theater under general or spinal anesthesia. Alternatively, spermatic cord block using lidocaine 2 percent with/without intravenous sedation can be performed in the outpatient setting, especially when percutaneous aspiration is intended.

6.3.3 Methods for Surgical Sperm Retrieval (Surgical Protocols)

6.3.3.1 Testicular Sperm Aspiration

Various modifications for TESA have been described. A simple aspiration cytology procedure can be performed using a 22 G butterfly needle, which is inserted into the testicular tissue while applying suction with a 20 ml syringe [3]. The aspirated fluid is then checked for sperm. Alternatively, needle aspiration biopsy (NAB) can be performed using an 18 G intravenous cannula inserted perpendicularly in the anterior surface of the testicle [7]. Once the cannula punctures the tunica albuginea, the needle is retrieved and the cannula is rotated 180 degrees a number of times. The cannula is then connected to a 20 ml syringe through an IV extension tube. While applying suction, the cannula is cautiously pulled and pushed within the testis until a column of testicular tissue can be visualized. The tubing is then clamped while under suction and the cannula is slowly pulled out of the testis. As the cannula emerges from the scrotal skin, a loop of seminiferous tubule will be observed, which can be grasped with microsurgical forceps, pulling additional tissue from the testis. This tissue, along with the contents of the cannula, are placed on a dry dish and inspected for the presence of sperm. The procedure can be repeated if the initial tissue is scanty or if no sperm are found. Finally, a tissue-cutting biopsy can also be performed to retrieve sperm percutaneously with the help of biopsy instruments (Tru-cut™ needle or Biopty™ gun) [31]. These needles are spring-activated, and are fired into the testis to retrieve a chip of tissue that can be analyzed for sperm. A short movie depicting the main steps of

37

the procedure can be found at www.youtube.com/watch?v=o9MgknYEzN0.

6.3.3.2 Conventional TESE

The open or cTESE procedure can be performed through a single incision along the scrotal midline raphe. Alternatively, some surgeons may prefer doing two separate transverse hemiscrotal incisions. The dartos muscle and tunica vaginalis are then incised and the testis is delivered from the wound. A tunica albuginea "window" is made using a no. 10 surgical scalpel. The emerging testicular tissue is cut with microsurgery scissors. Hemostasis is then achieved using low-current electrocautery and the tunical opening is closed with nonabsorbable sutures. The tunica vaginalis, dartos muscle, and scrotal skin are then closed with absorbable sutures. The testicular tissue is placed on a Petri dish containing sperm-friendly media and is sent to the lab for processing.

6.3.3.3 Single Seminiferous Tubule Biopsy

This procedure is a modification of cTESE [7]. The testis is delivered through a scrotal wall incision as described above. Using a 26 G needle, multiple punctures can be made through avascular areas of the testicular surface. These punctures are then dilated with the tip of a microforceps, allowing a loop of seminiferous tubule to pop out. This loop is then pulled with the microforceps and examined under the microscrope. The number of puncture holes is determined by the quantity of retrieved sperm and the quality of the seminiferous tubules. Since the holes are very small in size, no suturing is needed.

6.3.3.4 Micro-TESE [32]

After delivering the testis from the scrotal incision, the tunica albuginea is examined under low magnification (6–8×) and a large horizontal midline incision is made through an avascular plane. The midline edges of the tunica albuginea are then clamped with small mosquito forceps to help in bivalving the testicle along its equatorial plane. The testicular parenchyma is then explored using high magnification (16–25×), looking for dilated seminiferous tubules (which presumably are lined by germ cells and are likely to contain sperm). The dissection is carried out in a systematic fashion and dilated seminiferous tubules are retrieved using microforceps from superficial and deep layers of the testicular parenchyma. If the testicular parenchyma appears homogenous,

multiple random samples are retrieved from different areas of the testicular parenchyma. The samples are placed in a Petri dish containing sperm-friendly media and are sent to the laboratory for analysis. The tunica albuginea is then closed using nonabsorbable sutures in a running fashion. The remaining layers are closed with absorbable sutures. The wound is preferably injected with a local anesthetic (1 percent lidocaine) to reduce postoperative pain. A short movie depicting the main steps of the procedure can be found at www.brazjurol.com.br/videos/may_june_2013/Esteves_440_441video.htm [33].

6.3.4 Postoperative Care

All sperm retrieval procedures are performed in an outpatient setting and patients are generally discharged a few hours after the procedure. Patients are advised to apply scrotal ice packs and to stay in bed for the rest of the day of the procedure. After 24 hours, patients are advised to take a warm bath and wash the surgical site with soap and water. The incision should by dried with a sterile gauze and patients should be instructed to wear scrotal support for up to one week following surgery. Oral analgesics should be prescribed for 3–5 days after the procedure. Postoperative antibiotics are generally not required. Following TESA, patients can usually resume routine activities the following day; for open procedures, a sick leave of 3–7 days may be required. Strenuous physical activity and sexual intercourse should be avoided for up to 10 days following open procedures. Patients should be informed that swelling or ecchymosis of the surgical site can be expected to occur and will usually resolve within 1–2 weeks following surgery [34]. However, they should seek medical assistance if there is progressive pain, swelling, excessive bleeding, or discharge from the surgical site, or if they have a fever.

6.3.5 Complications of Testicular Sperm Retrieval

Persistent pain, infection, hydrocele, and hematoma are the most common complications that can occur following sperm retrieval procedures [4,5,35,36]. The complication rate varies according to the sperm retrieval technique performed. Since TESA is a blind technique, the risk of hematoma may be greater than for other procedures [36]. However, except for minor postoperative pain and swelling, no reports have indicated significant intra- or postoperative complications from TESA. Conventional TESE can have a detrimental effect on testicular function postoperatively, especially if large amounts of tissue were extracted [4,5,35]. Intratesticular hematomas were observed in up to 80 percent of patients undergoing scrotal ultrasound following testicular sperm extraction; however, this will often resolve spontaneously [36]. Micro-TESE is believed to offer a lower risk of complications as magnification will allow retrieval of less testicular tissue in addition to preservation of intratesticular blood supply. Nevertheless, transient reductions in serum testosterone are documented following micro-TESE and are believed to return to pre-surgical levels up to 12 months following the procedure [37].

6.4 Outcomes, Advantages, and Disadvantages of Different Surgical Sperm Retrieval Methods

6.4.1 Sperm Retrieval Outcomes

The testicular sperm retrieval rate for patients with NOA is influenced by a number of factors. While various predictors for testicular sperm retrieval have been recognized [38,39] and will be covered in detail in Chapter 10, the surgical procedure performed can significantly affect the sperm retrieval rate. The reported TESA retrieval rate ranges between 10 and 30 percent [36,40–44]. However, this rate increases to >65 percent in patients with previous positive TESA or with a testicular histopathology showing hypospermatogenesis [34,45]. The sperm retrieval rate with cTESE is about 50 percent [40], while that of micro-TESE ranges between 35 and 77 percent [34,46–53]. A systemic review by Deruyver et al. [54] compared the efficacy of micro-TESE to cTESE in men with NOA. The authors examined seven articles and reported a significantly higher sperm retrieval rate with micro-TESE (42.9–63 percent) in comparison to cTESE (16.7–45 percent). They also performed a sub-analysis of the sperm retrieval rate based on the histopathology result and observed a significantly better sperm retrieval rate with micro-TESE in patients with Sertoli-cell-only compared with cTESE. This result was echoed by another systematic review comparing three sperm retrieval methods: micro-TESE, TESA, and cTESE [40]. The results

indicate that in patients with Sertoli-cell-only, micro-TESE is better than cTESE, while cTESE is better than TESA. Bernie et al. [55] conducted a meta-analysis of 15 studies to compare the outcomes of micro-TESE, cTESE, and TESA. In a direct comparison, the sperm retrieval rate was 1.5 times higher in micro-TESE compared with cTESE (95 percent CI 1.4–1.6), while it was two times higher in cTESE compared with TESA (95 percent CI 1.8–2.2). Due to the heterogeneity of the conducted studies, none of these reviews was able to compare the pregnancy outcomes between the different sperm retrieval methods.

6.4.2 Number of Samples

The number of biopsies that can be sampled during the different sperm retrieval techniques has been a subject of debate. Studies have indicated that up to four biopsies can be obtained from each testicle with TESA or cTESE [56,57]. One study reported that the mean number of biopsies necessary to retrieve sperm from patients with maturation arrest or Sertoli-cell-only was 4.2 ± 4.5 and 2.8 ± 2.5, respectively [58]. Since SST and micro-TESE do not produce major trauma to the testicular tissue, anywhere between 10 and 15 biopsies can be taken [57].

6.4.3 Choice of Surgical Sperm Retrieval Technique

The ideal surgical sperm retrieval method is the one that offers the highest sperm retrieval rate together with the lowest complication rate. The expense of the procedure is also an important factor to consider as some procedures are much more expensive than others. Therefore, the choice of surgical procedure should be tailored to each case. A number of clinical factors can aid in selecting the most appropriate procedure for a given case. Testicular histopathology, if previously known, is a good example as TESA may be offered for men with hypospermatogenesis, while micro-TESE may be a better option for those with Sertoli-cell-only. Testicular volume is another example as reports have indicated that micro-TESE is better than cTESE in patients with testicular volume <10 ml [59]. Many authors have advocated a staged surgical approach to sperm retrieval, in which they would start first with TESA and progress to SST or micro-TESE if no sperm were found with percutaneous aspiration [57,60].

6.4.4 Advantages and Disadvantages of the Various Sperm Retrieval Techniques

Each surgical procedure has its advantages and disadvantages (Table 6.2). While percutaneous retrieval is a simpler and less invasive procedure, it offers lower retrieval rates, especially in men with Sertoli-cell-only histopathology. On the other hand, microsurgery allows the selective sampling of promising seminiferous tubules, resulting in better sperm retrieval rates and less testicular damage [61,62]. The higher number of retrieved sperm with micro-TESE allows for freezing and future ICSI treatments. With the advent of sperm freezing in small-volume carriers, including sperm vitrification, which yields satisfactory rates of sperm recovery and fertilization by ICSI, the use of methods that optimize this endpoint seems essential [61,63].

Another aspect to consider is the laboratory workload concerning processing and searching of the extracted tissue. The more precise the extraction process is, the less exhaustive the laboratory workload, thus reducing the risk of missing sperm in a "sea" of cells and debris. However, micro-TESE is more technically demanding and certainly more expensive than the other sperm retrieval procedures.

6.5 Conclusion

Testicular sperm retrieval is a well-established treatment used in a number of cases of male factor infertility in conjunction with ARTs. The highest sperm retrieval rate is obtained with micro-TESE, but this is at the expense of being an invasive and costly procedure that is preferably performed at centers of excellence. TESA is the least invasive but has the lowest retrieval rate and therefore may be performed in selected cases, such as those with previously successful TESA or histopathology showing hypospermatogenesis.

Table 6.2 Advantages and disadvantages of the different sperm retrieval techniques

Procedure	Sperm retrieval rate	Advantages	Disadvantages
Testicular sperm aspiration	10–30 percent [36,40–44]	Simple and quick procedure that does not require special instruments. No special training is required. The needle aspiration biopsy offers retrieval of testicular tissue that can be used for therapeutic as well as diagnostic purposes.	Blind procedure, therefore a tunical vessel may be injured, resulting in hematocele. Intratesticular hemorrhage may also occur due to the blind passage of the needle inside the testicular tissue. Scanty cellular material is retrieved.
Conventional testicular sperm extraction	50 percent [40]	Simple procedure that does not require special training. Yields a good amount of tissue.	Since no magnification is used, testicular vessels may be injured. Repeat open testicular sperm extractions may alter testicular function.
Single seminiferous tubule biopsy	–	Allows sufficient sampling of testicular tissue without performing a major incision to the tunica albuginea. Lower risk of testicular damage than conventional biopsy.	Open surgical procedure
Microsurgical testicular sperm extraction	35–77 percent [34,46–53]	Selective sampling of promising seminiferous tubules thereby minimizing testicular damage. Highest sperm retrieval rate since a large area of testicular parenchyma is inspected.	Requires microsurgery training. Time consuming. Longest recovery period.

References

1. Cocuzza M, Alvarenga C, Pagani R. The epidemiology and etiology of azoospermia. *Clinics (Sao Paulo)* 2013;68(Suppl. 1):15–26.

2. Devroey P, Liu J, Nagy Z, et al. Pregnancies after testicular sperm extraction and intracytoplasmic sperm injection in non-obstructive azoospermia. *Hum Reprod* 1995;10:1457–1460.

3. Craft I, Tsirigotis M. Simplified recovery, preparation and cryopreservation of testicular spermatozoa. *Hum Reprod* 1995;10:1623–1626.

4. Ron-El R, Strauss S, Friedler S, et al. Serial sonography and colour flow Doppler imaging following testicular and epididymal sperm extraction. *Hum Reprod* 1998;13:3390–3393.

5. Schlegel PN, Su LM. Physiological consequences of testicular sperm extraction. *Hum Reprod* 1997;12:1688–1692.

6. Schlegel PN, Li PS. Microdissection TESE: sperm retrieval in non-obstructive azoospermia. *Hum Reprod Update* 1998;4:439.

7. Shah RS. *Advanced Infertility Management.* Jaypee Brothers, New Delhi, 2002.

8. Temple-Smith PD, Southwick GJ, Yates CA, Trounson AO, de Kretser DM. Human pregnancy by in vitro fertilization (IVF) using sperm aspirated from the epididymis. *J In Vitro Fert Embryo Transf* 1985;2:119–122.

9. Esteves SC, Miyaoka R, Agarwal A. Sperm retrieval techniques for assisted reproduction. *Int Braz J Urol* 2011;37:570–583.

10. Sakkas D, Alvarez JG. Sperm DNA fragmentation: mechanisms of origin, impact on reproductive outcome, and analysis. *Fertil Steril* 2010;93:1027–1036.

11. Majzoub A, Agarwal A, Esteves SC. Sperm DNA fragmentation: a rationale for its clinical utility. *Transl Androl Urol* 2017;6:S455–S456.

12. Lewis SE, John Aitken R, Conner SJ, et al. The impact of sperm DNA damage in assisted conception and beyond: recent advances in diagnosis and treatment. *Reprod Biomed Online* 2013;27:325–337.

13. Leach M, Aitken RJ, Sacks G. Sperm DNA fragmentation abnormalities in men from couples with a history of recurrent miscarriage. *Aust N Z J Obstet Gynaecol* 2015;55:379–383.

14. Jin J, Pan C, Fei Q, et al. Effect of sperm DNA fragmentation on the clinical outcomes for in vitro fertilization and intracytoplasmic sperm injection in women with different ovarian reserves. *Fertil Steril* 2015;103:910–916.

15. Majzoub A, Agarwal A, Esteves SC. Sperm DNA fragmentation for the evaluation of male infertility: clinical algorithms. *Transl Androl Urol* 2017;6:S405–S408.

16. Agarwal A, Cho CL, Majzoub A, Esteves SC. The Society for Translational Medicine: clinical practice guidelines for sperm DNA fragmentation testing in male infertility. *Transl Androl Urol* 2017;6:S720–S733.

17. Wright C, Milne S, Leeson H. Sperm DNA damage caused by oxidative stress: modifiable clinical, lifestyle and nutritional factors in male infertility. *Reprod Biomed Online* 2014;28:684–703.

18. Sakkas D, Mariethoz E, Manicardi G, et al. Origin of DNA damage in ejaculated human spermatozoa. *Rev Reprod* 1999;4:31–37.

19. Ni K, Steger K, Yang H, et al. A comprehensive investigation of sperm DNA damage and oxidative stress injury in infertile patients with subclinical, normozoospermic, and astheno/oligozoospermic clinical varicocoele. *Andrology* 2016;4:816–824.

20. Moustafa MH, Sharma RK, Thornton J, et al. Relationship between ROS production, apoptosis and DNA denaturation in spermatozoa from patients examined for infertility. *Hum Reprod* 2004;19:129–138.

21. Majzoub A, Arafa M, Mahdi M, et al. Oxidation-reduction potential and sperm DNA fragmentation, and their associations with sperm morphological anomalies amongst fertile and infertile men. *Arab J Urol* 2018;16:87–95.

22. Greco E, Scarselli F, Iacobelli M, et al. Efficient treatment of infertility due to sperm DNA damage by ICSI with testicular spermatozoa. *Hum Reprod* 2005;20:226–230.

23. Moskovtsev SI, Jarvi K, Mullen JB, et al. Testicular spermatozoa have statistically significantly lower DNA damage compared with ejaculated spermatozoa in patients with unsuccessful oral antioxidant treatment. *Fertil Steril* 2010;93:1142–1146.

24. Esteves SC, Sanchez-Martin F, Sanchez-Martin P, Schneider DT, Gosalvez J. Comparison of reproductive outcome in oligozoospermic men with high sperm DNA fragmentation undergoing intracytoplasmic sperm injection with ejaculated and testicular sperm. *Fertil Steril* 2015;104:1398–1405.

25. Esteves SC, Roque M, Bradley CK, Garrido N. Reproductive outcomes of testicular versus ejaculated sperm for intracytoplasmic sperm injection among men with high levels of

DNA fragmentation in semen: systematic review and meta-analysis. *Fertil Steril* 2017;108:456–467.

26. Mehta A, Bolyakov A, Schlegel PN, Paduch DA. Higher pregnancy rates using testicular sperm in men with severe oligospermia. *Fertil Steril* 2015;104:1382–1387.

27. Esteves SC, Roque M, Garrido N. Use of testicular sperm for intracytoplasmic sperm injection in men with high sperm DNA fragmentation: a SWOT analysis. *Asian J Androl* 2018;20:1–8.

28. Ketabchi AA. Intracytoplasmic sperm injection outcomes with freshly ejaculated sperms and testicular or epididymal sperm extraction in patients with idiopathic cryptozoospermia. *Nephrourol Mon* 2016;8:e41375.

29. Ben-Ami I, Raziel A, Strassburger D, et al. Intracytoplasmic sperm injection outcome of ejaculated versus extracted testicular spermatozoa in cryptozoospermic men. *Fertil Steril* 2013;99:1867–1871.

30. Kang YN, Hsiao YW, Chen CY, Wu CC. Testicular sperm is superior to ejaculated sperm for ICSI in cryptozoospermia: an update systematic review and meta-analysis. *Sci Rep* 2018;8:7874.

31. Morey AF, Deshon GE, Jr., Rozanski TA, Dresner ML. Technique of biopty gun testis needle biopsy. *Urology* 1993;42:325–326.

32. Schlegel PN. Nonobstructive azoospermia: a revolutionary surgical approach and results. *Semin Reprod Med* 2009;27:165–170.

33. Esteves SC. Microdissection testicular sperm extraction (micro-TESE) as a sperm acquisition method for men with nonobstructive azoospermia seeking fertility: operative and laboratory aspects. *Int Braz J Urol* 2013;39:440.

34. Esteves SC, Agarwal A. *Sperm Retrieval Techniques.* Cambridge University Press, Cambridge, 2011.

35. Ramasamy R, Yagan N, Schlegel PN. Structural and functional changes to the testis after conventional versus microdissection testicular sperm extraction. *Urology* 2005;65:1190–1194.

36. Carpi A, Menchini Fabris FG, Palego P, et al. Fine-needle and large-needle percutaneous aspiration biopsy of testicles in men with nonobstructive azoospermia: safety and diagnostic performance. *Fertil Steril* 2005;83:1029–1033.

37. Komori K, Tsujimura A, Miura H, et al. Serial follow-up study of serum testosterone and antisperm antibodies in patients with non-obstructive azoospermia after conventional or microdissection testicular sperm extraction. *Int J Androl* 2004;27:32–36.

38. Xu T, Peng L, Lin X, Li J, Xu W. Predictors for successful sperm retrieval of salvage microdissection testicular sperm extraction (TESE) following failed TESE in nonobstructive azoospermia patients. *Andrologia* 2017;49. doi: 10.1111/and.12642.

39. Cissen M, Meijerink AM, D'Hauwers KW, et al. Prediction model for obtaining spermatozoa with testicular sperm extraction in men with non-obstructive azoospermia. *Hum Reprod* 2016;31:1934–1941.

40. Donoso P, Tournaye H, Devroey P. Which is the best sperm retrieval technique for non-obstructive azoospermia? A systematic review. *Hum Reprod Update* 2007;13:539–549.

41. Carpi A, Sabanegh E, Mechanick J. Controversies in the management of nonobstructive azoospermia. *Fertil Steril* 2009;91:963–970.

42. Ezeh UI, Moore HD, Cooke ID. A prospective study of multiple needle biopsies versus a single open biopsy for testicular sperm extraction in men with non-obstructive azoospermia. *Hum Reprod* 1998;13:3075–3080.

43. Hauser R, Yogev L, Paz G, et al. Comparison of efficacy of two techniques for testicular sperm retrieval in nonobstructive azoospermia: multifocal testicular sperm extraction versus multifocal testicular sperm aspiration. *J Androl* 2006;27:28–33.

44. Friedler S, Raziel A, Strassburger D, et al. Testicular sperm retrieval by percutaneous fine needle sperm aspiration compared with testicular sperm extraction by open biopsy in men with non-obstructive azoospermia. *Hum Reprod* 1997;12:1488–1493.

45. Esteves SC, Verza S, Prudencio C, Seol B. Sperm retrieval rates (SRR) in nonobstructive azoospermia (NOA) are related to testicular histopathology results but not to the etiology of azoospermia. *Fertil Steril* 2010;94:S132.

46. Schlegel PN. Testicular sperm extraction: microdissection improves sperm yield with minimal tissue excision. *Hum Reprod* 1999;14:131–135.

47. Schiff JD, Palermo GD, Veeck LL, et al. Success of testicular sperm extraction [corrected] and intracytoplasmic sperm injection in men with Klinefelter syndrome. *J Clin Endocrinol Metab* 2005;90:6263–6367.

48. Turunc T, Gul U, Haydardedeoglu B, et al. Conventional testicular sperm extraction combined with the microdissection technique in nonobstructive azoospermic patients: a prospective comparative study. *Fertil Steril* 2010;94:2157–2160.

49. Silber SJ. Microsurgical TESE and the distribution of spermatogenesis in non-obstructive azoospermia. *Hum Reprod* 2000;15:2278–2284.

50. Okada H, Dobashi M, Yamazaki T, et al. Conventional versus microdissection testicular sperm extraction for nonobstructive azoospermia. *J Urol* 2002;168:1063–1067.

51. Tsujimura A. Microdissection testicular sperm extraction: prediction, outcome, and complications. *Int J Urol* 2007;14:883–889.

52. Chan PT, Palermo GD, Veeck LL, Rosenwaks Z, Schlegel PN. Testicular sperm extraction combined with intracytoplasmic sperm injection in the treatment of men with persistent azoospermia postchemotherapy. *Cancer* 2001;92:1632–1637.

53. Raman JD, Schlegel PN. Testicular sperm extraction with intracytoplasmic sperm injection is successful for the treatment of nonobstructive azoospermia associated with cryptorchidism. *J Urol* 2003;170:1287–1290.

54. Deruyver Y, Vanderschueren D, Van der Aa F. Outcome of microdissection TESE compared with conventional TESE in non-obstructive azoospermia: a systematic review. *Andrology* 2014;2:20–24.

55. Bernie AM, Mata DA, Ramasamy R, Schlegel PN. Comparison of microdissection testicular sperm extraction, conventional testicular sperm extraction, and testicular sperm aspiration for nonobstructive azoospermia: a systematic review and meta-analysis. *Fertil Steril* 2015;104:1099–1103.

56. Altay B, Hekimgil M, Cikili N, Turna B, Soydan S. Histopathological mapping of open testicular biopsies in patients with unobstructive azoospermia. *BJU Int* 2001;87:834–837.

57. Shah RS. Surgical sperm retrieval: techniques and their indications. *Indian J Urol* 2011;27:102–109.

58. Tournaye H, Liu J, Nagy PZ, et al. Correlation between testicular histology and outcome after intracytoplasmic sperm injection using testicular spermatozoa. *Hum Reprod* 1996;11:127–132.

59. Mulhall JP, Ghaly SW, Aviv N, Ahmed A. The utility of optical loupe magnification for testis sperm extraction in men with nonobstructive azoospermia. *J Androl* 2005;26:178–181.

60. Esteves SC, Miyaoka R, Orosz JE, Agarwal A. An update on sperm retrieval techniques for azoospermic males. *Clinics (Sao Paulo)* 2013;68(1):99–110.

61. Esteves SC. Clinical management of infertile men with nonobstructive azoospermia. *Asian J Androl* 2015;17:459–470.

62. Miyaoka R, Orosz JE, Achermann AP, Esteves SC. Methods of surgical sperm extraction and implications for assisted reproductive technology success. *Panminerva Med* 2019;61:164–177.

63. Esteves SC. Novel concepts in male factor infertility: clinical and laboratory perspectives. *J Assist Reprod Genet* 2016;33:1319–1335.

Surgical and Nonsurgical Sperm Retrieval Techniques in Patients with Ejaculatory Dysfunctions

Omer Raheem, Mohamed Adnan, and Laith M. Alzweri

7.1 Introduction

Ejaculatory dysfunction (EjD) is the most common sexual dysfunction in men [1,2]. The spectrum of EjD covers premature ejaculation (PE), delayed ejaculation (DE), retrograde ejaculation (RE), and a complete inability to ejaculate, also known as anejaculation (AE) [3]. Moreover, EjD can also lead to low-volume ejaculate, which may be a contributing male infertility factor in men seeking fatherhood. Several surgical and nonsurgical sperm retrieval methods are used to obtain sperm from the epididymis and/or testes in men with ejaculatory dysfunctions (Table 7.1). The selection of technique depends on the clinical scenario and feasibility.

7.1.1 Normal Ejaculatory Mechanism

The two important phases of normal ejaculation are emission and expulsion. These processes are mediated by somatic, sympathetic, parasympathetic, afferent, and efferent fibers. The first phase of ejaculation is emission, which consists of a peristaltic contraction of the smooth muscles in the seminal tract until the ejaculate reaches the prostate. Ejaculate is then deposited into the posterior urethra. The latter phase, expulsion, happens when the semen is forcefully and rapidly advanced through the urethra and then out the penis. Adequate propulsion of semen necessitates synchronized relaxation of the external urinary sphincter with accompanying bladder neck closure, rhythmic contractions of the striated muscles of the bulbospongiosus muscles and the pelvic floor [4]. The ejaculation process can be triggered in several ways, such as influences from various cortical stimuli as well as tactile stimulation of the glans penis [5].

7.1.2 Pathophysiology

Multiple neurotransmitter systems at supraspinal and spinal regions are involved in the regulation of the ejaculatory reflex. A wide range of neurotransmitters, including dopamine, nitric oxide, oxytocin, adrenaline, c-aminobutyric acid, 5-hydroxytryptamine (5-HT), serotonin, and acetylcholine have a role, particularly in the central nervous system (CNS) [6–8]. The neurotransmitter that is most studied in the neurophysiology of ejaculation is 5-HT [9]. There are 14 different 5-HT receptor subtypes reported so far, each having a different function and neuroanatomical location [10]. The 5-HT_{1a} somatodendritic autoreceptors that are present in the medullary and mesencephalic raphe nuclei are responsible for diminishing 5-HT release into the synapse via a negative feedback mechanism and decreasing ejaculatory latency [11, 12]. The 5-HT_{1b} and 5-HT_{2c} receptors, in contrast to the 5-HT_{1a} autoreceptors, are located in the postsynaptic membrane, and they have been shown to extend ejaculatory latency. It is likely that the mechanism behind ejaculatory disorders is the change in levels of 5-HT or altered 5-HT receptor sensitivity in the ejaculatory regulating centers of the CNS [12].

7.1.3 Implications of EjD on Fecundity

Ejaculatory dysfunction is one of the major causes of male infertility and is a serious problem in young patients. Therefore, therapeutic management of EjD has become very crucial for couples wishing for a baby. Semen analysis is a crucial exam for the diagnosis of male infertility. An adequate volume of ejaculate is necessary to carry the male gametes into the reproductive tract of the female [13]. The 2010 World Health Organization (WHO) criteria consider 1.5 ml semen volume as the lower reference limit and ≥ 15 million sperm/ml is regarded as normal [14]. Ejaculatory dysfunction may impact the semen quality parameters by reducing volume, sperm count, and motility.

Retrograde ejaculation and anejaculation are common causes of EjD. The etiology and treatment

Table 7.1 Summary of the medical and surgical treatment options in patients with concomitant infertility and ejaculatory dysfunction

Type	Definition	Causes	Diagnosis	Treatments
Anejaculation/ anorgasmia (AE)	Complete failure to attain emission despite adequate stimulation.	Anatomic, genetic, endocrine, infectious, and neurobiological factors, or it may be drug-induced	Post-orgasmic urinalysis: complete absence of antegrade ejaculation and a non-viscous, sperm-negative, and fructose-negative semen	**Medical treatment** Behavioral: psychosexual counseling Pharmacological: cabergoline, alpha adrenoceptor agonists (pseudoephedrine) Procedural: penile vibratory stimulation (PVS), Electroejaculation (EEJ) **Surgical treatment** Testicular sperm aspiration (TESA) Testicular sperm extraction (TESE) Epididymal sperm aspiration (percutaneous or microsurgical):
Retrograde ejaculation (RE)	Insufficient bladder neck resistance to the high pressures yielded by the ischiocavernosus and bulbospongiosus muscles during ejaculation, causing redirection of semen into the bladder	Medication (tamsulosin), surgical (transurethral resection of the prostate), retroperitoneal surgical resection and complications of diabetes	Urinalysis obtained immediately postcoital or post-orgasm with >10–15 sperm per high power field validates the presence of RE	**Medical treatment** Pharmacological: pseudoephedrine; alpha agonists; Imipramine, (tricyclic antidepressant) **Surgical treatment** Young–Dees procedure: Abrahams procedure: Alloplastic spermatocele: TESA TESE Epididymal sperm aspiration (percutaneous or microsurgical):
Premature ejaculation (PE)	Lifelong PE: ejaculation that always or nearly always occurs prior to or within about 1 minute of vaginal penetration Acquired PE: clinically significant reduction in latency time after penetration, often to about 3 minutes or less	Higher levels of education, presence of social phobia, relational difficulties, psychological factors such as stress, depression, guilt	Validated questionnaire: premature ejaculation profile (PEP), premature ejaculation diagnostic tool, or index of premature ejaculation if the patient has concomitant erectile dysfunction	**Medical treatment** Behavioral: psychosexual counseling Pharmacological: selective serotonin reuptake inhibitors (SSRIs), phosphodiesterase 5 inhibitors (PDE5), and eutectic mixture of prilocaine and lidocaine Topical agents (Promescent®) **Surgical treatment** Penile hypoanesthesia via hyaluronic acid gel glans penis augmentation Selective dorsal nerve neurotomy

of RE and AE in male infertility have been comparatively well studied [15, 16]. Men who have AE or RE in their reproductive phase due to any reason can lead to infertility. Spinal cord injury (SCI) is the major cause of neurogenic AE. Psychogenic erections need the supraspinal input to the cord with intact thoracolumbar roots, and therefore they are frequently lost with injuries to the thoracic spinal cord [17]. Therefore, some men with SCI can initiate reflexogenic erections. However, they cannot preserve them due to the absence of psychogenic erections [18]. Diabetes complications are also responsible for RE, with one series describing a prevalence of 32 percent [19]. Surgery and instrumentation are also reported as important factors causing AE. Both often lead to an incompetent bladder neck, with most men experiencing RE after transurethral resection of the prostate [20]. Alpha-receptor antagonists given for lower urinary tract symptoms can also cause RE [21].

7.1.4 Prevalence and Pregnancy Outcomes

Ejaculatory problems have been reported by 74.3 percent, 54.9 percent, and 30.1 percent of men aged 70–80, 60–69, and 50–59 years, respectively.[22]. Retrograde ejaculation contributes to 0.3–2 percent of male infertility [23, 24], whereas PE impacts up to 30 percent of the adult male population and is regarded as the most common sexual disorder in men [1]. Ejaculatory dysfunction-related infertility is one of the most serious problems for men seeking fatherhood. Erectile dysfunction is an important post-testicular cause of male infertility, and there have been major advances in our understanding of this disorder. However, if sexual intercourse is attained successfully without any ejaculate, the female partner will not be able to conceive. Hence, the establishment of management of EjD is increasingly important for couples wishing to conceive a child. The therapeutic approach to EjD-related male factor infertility is indicated when EjD is the main reason for having no children and if EjD is also accompanied by worsening of semen quality.

7.2 Anejaculation/Anorgasmia

Anejaculation is identified as a complete absence of ejaculation despite adequate stimulation. Men commonly discontinue sexual interaction given exhaustion, partner request, or irritation [25]. An orgasm is defined as the climax of sexual arousal which is felt

throughout the body, whereas ejaculation involves the release of sperm carrying fluid following sexual activity. There is a difference between orgasm and ejaculation, but most men will present with a complaint of combined inability to orgasm or ejaculate. Total AE is the situation in which the man is unable to ejaculate semen consciously with normal orgasm, either by masturbation or during intercourse. Anejaculation covers complete RE, anorgasmia, or failure of emission. Complete RE can occur because of any of the causes of AE, whereas DE is mostly due to a neurological reason with disruption of sympathetic nerves or output.

7.2.1 Prevalence

Anejaculation, anorgasmia, and DE are among the uncommon and least understood male sexual health dysfunctions. The estimated prevalence of AE/DE is approximately 1–4 percent of the male population [26–28].

7.2.2 Causes and Pathophysiology

Anejaculation is caused by anatomic, genetic, endocrine, infectious, and neurobiological factors, or it may be drug-induced. It may also be caused by psychosocial, relationship, or psychosexual problems. Any drug, medical disease, congenital abnormality, or surgical procedure that interferes with either the peripheral control or central control of ejaculation that includes sympathetic nerve supply to the seminal vesicles, bladder neck, vas deferens, or prostate, as well as the somatic efferent nerve supply to the pelvic region, can lead to AE and anorgasmia. From a medication standpoint, the most well-known drugs are from the antidepressant class (SSRIs), which enhance the amount of circulating 5-HT, an ejaculatory inhibitor [29]. Medical diseases include hypothyroidism and alcoholic or diabetic neuropathy [30], even cerebro-vascular accident (CVA) related to the impairment of orgasm [31], and low testosterone [32]. Anatomically, surgical procedures such as prostatectomy, transurethral resection of the prostate (TURP), bladder neck incision, retroperitoneal lymph node dissection (RPLND), or other pelvic or colorectal surgery and SCIs, which can damage pelvic nerves, may also cause DE [33, 34]. Patients who use serotonergic antidepressants frequently describe sexual dysfunction. Around seven-fold higher risk for AE has been observed in SSRI users [35]. The significant heterogeneity in the presentation of SSRI-related sexual dysfunction and its occurrence may indicate underlying genetic factors [36]. Aging can also lead to decreased penile sensitivity, which has been attributed to possible degenerative age-related or ultrastructural changes in the penile receptors [37,38], ultimately leading to progressive axonal sensory loss [39, 40].

7.2.3 Diagnosis

Diagnostic clues to AE are the complete absence of antegrade ejaculation and a non-viscous, sperm-negative, and fructose-negative post-orgasmic urinalysis [41].

7.2.4 Treatment

7.2.4.1 Nonsurgical: Behavioral-Psychosexual Therapy

Given the large psychosocial component of AE, referral to a sexual therapist can be important to assess and treat behavioral, relational, or psychological issues. Psychosexual therapy can be specifically helpful in primary inhibited orgasm [42] when it is not due to a medical disease, surgical side effects, or medication.

7.2.4.2 Medical

Cabergoline is a potent dopamine receptor agonist. It is thought to promote ejaculation by increasing dopamine neurotransmission. Cabergoline (0.5 mg twice/week) was tested for the treatment of anorgasmic men who were non-responders to the treatment for testosterone deficiency [43]. The authors found that 25 percent of men had improved orgasmic function. Bupropion (150 mg daily), which acts via blocking the reuptake of both norepinephrine and dopamine, is used as an agent in depressed men when SSRIs cause AE [44]. Testosterone replacement has been assessed as a potential treatment for anejaculation. However, exogenous testosterone treatment is contraindicated in men seeking fertility as it can change the natural balance of the hypothalamic–pituitary–gonadal axis, resulting in impaired spermatogenesis and possibly azoospermia. Other alternative treatments in EjD patients are electroejaculation (EEJ) [45] or penile vibratory stimulation (PVS) [46], especially for the treatment of AE in patients with SCI. An alpha-agonist, such as ephedrine (15–60 mg), pseudoephedrine (60–120 mg), imipramine (25–75 mg), and midodrine (7.5–22.5 mg max.), can be considered if an anejaculatory male is trying to achieve fertility

[47]. Alpha agonists may change AE to RE, which helps in sperm retrieval from the urine.

7.2.4.3 Penile Vibratory Stimulation

In PVS, a vibrator is placed against the penis and then supraphysiological mechanical stimulation is applied to induce ejaculation. Although PVS is a comparatively safe and low-cost alternative, it needs at least one intact lumbosacral spinal cord segment (above T10) [48]. There are various methods of applying PVS: (1) placing one FertiCare personal device (Multicept, Denmark) to the frenulum or dorsum of the glans penis; (2) placing the glans penis between two FertiCare devices; and (3) placing the glans penis between two vibrating surfaces of a Viberect-X3 device (Reflexonic LLC, Frederick, USA). The above devices are specific vibrators available for patients with SCI. These vibrators have the capacity to deliver an amplitude of 2.5 mm, also known as "high-amplitude vibrators." It has been found that these high-amplitude vibrators can significantly increase ejaculatory success rate compared to lower-amplitude vibrators (96 percent vs. 32 percent ejaculatory success rate, respectively) [49].

7.2.4.4 Electroejaculation

Electroejaculation is a technique to collect semen to analyze and potentially freeze or store sperm or immediately process semen for artificial insemination. This technique was developed originally by veterinary specialists. During the procedure, a mild electric current is utilized to induce an ejaculation under anesthesia or in the absence of anesthesia (for men with SCI). Electroejaculation permits men unable to ejaculate to conceive a child. Several conditions lead to AE, including SCI, multiple sclerosis, radical abdominal and pelvic surgeries, and diabetes. Electroejaculation may be successful in obtaining ejaculate from men with all types of SCI, and from men who do not have deficit of major elements of the ejaculatory reflex arc. Any other situations that impact the ejaculatory mechanism of the peripheral and/or central nervous system, including surgical nerve injury, may also be treated successfully with EEJ.

Electroejaculation is generally performed transrectally (rectal probe EEJ). The probe is placed in the dorsal lithotomy position or lateral decubitus. Antegrade ejaculation is collected during stimulation, and the retrograde fraction is captured via postprocedural catheterization. Patients are usually prepared through emptying the bladder and inserting a sperm-friendly medium (solution) into the bladder prior to the procedure. Many men (including some men with SCI) may need general anesthesia for EEJ due to significant discomfort and potentially severe side effects, mainly originating from autonomic dysreflexia.

Special care must be taken during this procedure to monitor rectal temperature in order to prevent rectal mucosal burns. Anoscopy is generally performed immediately before and after EEJ. Monitoring of the rectal mucosa in this manner is highly recommended. This technique is also recommended for AE patients who failed to ejaculate with PVS and those taking sedatives and narcotics, males with past pelvic surgery/trauma or peripheral neuropathy, and men with significant genital, perineal, or pelvic edema.

7.2.5 Surgical Techniques

The most common surgical procedure employed for the management of EjD-related infertility is known as surgical sperm retrieval (SSR). This is based on the extreme progression in the techniques of ART (intracytoplasmic sperm injection, *in vitro* fertilization [IVF], sperm cryopreservation). Patients with RE or AE who fail to ejaculate or have insufficient spermatozoa within ejaculates under nonsurgical treatments could be directed for SSR. Anejaculation is not usually linked to defective spermatogenesis. Therefore, testicular sperm aspiration (TESA) and extraction (TESE) are routinely used SSR procedures. Testicular sperm aspiration is a needle aspirate collected from seminiferous tubules which contains both immature and mature sperm, both motile and non-motile. It is easy to perform without oral or conscious sedation. A study reported 61.4 percent pregnancy rate using TESA with cryopreservation [50]. The TESE procedure requires making a small incision in the testis to examine the presence of sperm in the tubules. It is usually performed in the operating room with sedation, but can also be performed with local anesthetic alone. A study demonstrated that the pregnancy outcome was 86.5 percent using this technique for couples in whom the male partner was suffering from EjD [51].

7.3 Retrograde Ejaculation

Retrograde ejaculation is specified as substantial propulsion of seminal fluid from seminal vesicles into the bladder via the posterior urethra. It can occur because of structural or functional disruption of the ejaculation process, such as insufficient bladder neck resistance to the high pressures yielded by the ischio-cavernosus and bulbospongiosus muscles during ejaculation, causing backward redirection of semen into the bladder [52]. The function of the bladder neck can be impacted by post-traumatic anatomical disruption via surgery (i.e., TURP) or pelvic fracture, or through processes modifying the nerve input to the sphincter. It can also be affected by alteration into the neuroreceptors within the bladder neck. Therefore, RE can either be partial or complete based on the severity of the neurological injury. Surgical injury to the nerves affecting the ejaculatory function is also a risk of RE, with the most common being spine, colorectal, and retroperitoneal surgeries [53, 54]. However, the introduction of the nerve-sparing RPLND technique has made this pillar of testicular cancer therapy less detrimental to patients' ejaculatory function [55]. Retrograde ejaculation is the most common cause for EjD in the absence of antegrade ejaculation, and contributes to 0.3–2 percent of male infertility [23,24].

7.3.1 Prevalence

Retrograde ejaculation is both under-recognized and common in diabetic men, with one study reporting a prevalence of 32 percent [19]. It is responsible for only 0.3–2 percent of infertility, despite being a common type of ejaculatory dysfunction [47]. Also, RE was the observed cause in 18 percent of azoospermic men; however, as a source of infertility it was only implicated in 0.7 percent [4,56].

7.3.2 Causes and Pathophysiology

Various medications, such as alpha-receptor antagonists (e.g., tamsulosin), antipsychotics, antidepressants, and other sympatholytics, surgical procedures (TURP), and complications of diabetic peripheral neuropathy can cause RE. It has been observed that the incidence is likely rising as an effect of increasing rates of diabetes, bladder neck surgery for malignancies, and the use of α-receptor antagonists [57]. Surgical injury to the nerves influencing ejaculatory function also pose the risk of RE, with the most common being spinal surgery, retroperitoneal and colorectal and other radical pelvic surgeries [53,54]. Moreover, the most common reason for RE is a history of RPLND for the treatment of testicular cancer, especially in patients in infertility clinics. Notably, the evolution of the surgical template for RPLND has resulted in important modifications to save the ejaculatory functions [13,15].

7.3.3 Diagnosis

Diagnosis is by urinalysis performed on a urine sample that is obtained immediately after ejaculation. In cases of RE, the specimen will carry an abnormal level of sperm. Anejaculation can often be confused with RE, especially in case of orgasmic AE. They share some fundamental etiology – urinalysis is employed to distinguish between them. A physical exam of the genitals is also used to ensure that there are no anatomical abnormalities. The urine will be assessed for the presence of semen. If there are no sperm in the urine, it may be due to injury to the prostate as a result of prior radiation therapy or surgery. The most useful assessment of RE is the evaluation of postcoital urine samples or post-orgasm. A finding of $>10–15$ sperm per high power field validates the presence of RE [58]. The post-ejaculatory urine sample is collected from patients undergoing a semen analysis. The sample is investigated for the number, morphology, and presence of sperm.

7.3.4 Pregnancy Outcomes

Jefferys et al. have examined several studies using a variety of artificial insemination techniques with the obtained sperm (IVF, ICSI, and intrauterine insemination [IUI]). Overall, the pregnancy rate per cycle was 15 percent, and the live birth rate was 14 percent [47]. The pregnancy rate per cycle was increased to 44.4 percent after successful treatment of RE [59].

7.3.5 Treatment

7.3.5.1 Nonsurgical Techniques (Medical)

Treatment of pharmacologic RE requires discontinuing the offending drug if desirable and medically safe. For other etiologies of RE, medical therapies are first-line in spite of the lack of robust studies supporting their use. Alpha agonists such as pseudoephedrine have been utilized off-label to stimulate more robust bladder neck contraction. In a recent prospective trial of 20 men with complete or partial RE dosed with 60 mg pseudoephedrine every 6 h the day before semen analysis and two additional doses on the day

of semen analysis, 70 percent of patients showed improvement in semen parameters such as ejaculate volume, percentage of total spermatozoa in urine, total sperm count in antegrade ejaculate, percentage of total motility, and total motile count in antegrade ejaculate [60]. The tricyclic antidepressant imipramine (25 mg twice/day) has also been employed alone and in combination with an alpha-agonist, with mild success [47,61].

7.3.5.2 Surgical Techniques

Sperm retrieval can be done by nonsurgical methods in certain conditions. In men with persistent RE or if sperm within antegrade ejaculates are not enough for artificial insemination despite medical therapy, the recovery of retrograde ejaculates from the bladder via catheterization is possible [62]. The process starts with complete catheterization of the bladder and then instillation of an insemination buffer medium into the bladder. This step can derogate possible damaging effects of urine on retrograde ejaculate. The catheter is then removed. After collecting the antegrade ejaculate, the bladder is catheterized again. Surgical intervention utilizing collagen injection at the bladder neck has been reported with variable success rates; it has not been established as a treatment modality [63].

Surgical procedures for patients with RE for the restitution of normal ejaculation are the Young–Dees operation [64] and the Abrahams technique [65]. All other surgical techniques that can be used in patients with RE or AE in whom spermatozoa cannot be retrieved otherwise are aimed solely at sperm recovery (e.g., Wagenknecht alloplastic spermatocele [66–68], Brindley reservoir [69], recovery of epididymal microsurgical vas deferens aspiration [70], or epydimal and testicular spermatozoa [MESA/TESA/TESE][71] for ART). Notably, these procedures are not routinely performed for patients with PE due to their invasiveness and complication rates, which are considerably higher than for traditional sperm retrieval procedures.

The Young–Dees operation is a type of bladder neck reconstruction to change RE into antegrade ejaculation. It could be the appropriate option for bladder neck incompetence at the time of ejaculation. The procedure decreases the caliber of the bladder neck, increases the deep urethra proximally, and supports the new bladder neck with trigonal muscle. This procedure can be considered when treatments such as sympathomimetic drugs and sperm retrieval from the urine for insemination are not successful. The rate of success for this operation is 80 percent [72]. The Abrahams technique was specifically used for patients with RE following Y-V plasty of the bladder during childhood. The procedure involves a transvesical approach to rebuilding the internal sphincteric mechanism.

Wagenknect et al. [67, 68] generated alloplastic spermatocele from a silicone elastomer. An alloplastic spermatocele is a container for sperm. This container can be punctured to collect the contents, which can be used to artificially inseminate the female partner. This is an effective method to retrieve fertile sperm from men suffering from EjD. The patient group includes men who are suffering from uncorrectable obstruction of the ejaculatory ducts, congenital hypoplasia or aplasia of the vas deferens, and inability to ejaculate for psychological or physiological reasons. The Brindley reservoir is another type of container used for the collection of sperm. It is sutured to the vas deferens for sperm retrieval and assisted conception.

Microsurgical epididymal sperm aspiration (MESA) requires dissection of the epididymis under the operating microscope and incision of an epididymal tubule. Fluid spills from the tubule and pools in the epididymal bed. This fluid is then collected. In TESA, spermatozoa are aspirated from a testicle by inserting a needle and aspirating tissue and fluid with negative pressure. Lastly, TESE is a surgical biopsy of the testis, which can be done with the aid of a microscope to enhance the sperm retrieval rate. The aspirated/biopsied tissue is then treated in the embryology laboratory and the sperm cells are extracted to use for assisted conception.

7.4 Premature Ejaculation

Premature ejaculation is an incompletely understood condition that impacts up to 30 percent of the adult male population and is regarded as the most common sexual disorder in men [1]. The vagueness surrounding PE is partially due to the challenges associated with accurately defining and classifying the clinical condition among patients [73]. Based on the International Society for Sexual Medicine (ISSM) 2014 criteria[74], PE can be classified into two categories: lifelong PE is defined as the ejaculation that always or nearly always occurs prior to or within about one minute of vaginal penetration; acquired PE is defined as the clinically significant reduction

in latency time after penetration, often to about three minutes or less. Premature ejaculation does not directly lead to infertility, but coexists in around one-third of ED patients [75]. Moreover, PE due to hypoactive sexual desire may be an outcome of hidden hypogonadism that extends to reduced semen quality [76]. Premature ejaculation is mainly a sexual dysfunction and unlikely to be a major contributing factor to male infertility.

7.4.1 Prevalence

Premature ejaculation is one of the most common male sexual disorders and has been estimated to occur in around 4–39 percent of men in the general population [2,77–79].

7.4.2 Causes

Higher levels of education, the presence of social phobia, and relational difficulties such as divorce appear to increase the risk of PE [80,81]. Anxiety has also been described as a cause of PE in multiple studies and is suggested in the traditional knowledge of sexual medicine as its most likely cause [82,83]. Sexual repression (blocked or bottled-up sexual feelings), stress, unrealistic expectations about sex, temporary depression, guilt, relationship problems, and a lack of confidence are also factors responsible for PE.

7.4.3 Pathophysiology

Hypersensitivity of the $5-HT_{1A}$ and/or hyposensitivity of the $5-HT_{2C}$ receptors have been indicated as a possible explanation for lifelong PE [84,85]. Men with probable $5-HT_{2C}$ receptor hyposensitivity and with low 5-HT neurotransmission may have their ejaculatory threshold genetically adjusted to a lower point and ejaculate quickly with minimal stimulation. Several authors have proposed the possibility that excessive and controlling concerns about sexual performance, potential sexual failure, and high levels of anxiety might distract a man from recognizing the prodromal sensations that precede ejaculatory inevitability and monitoring his level of arousal [86]. Premature ejaculation clearly has an effect on the mind of its sufferer, as well as their partners.

7.4.4 Diagnosis

A physical exam can be used to measure the risk factors and causal diseases but is not compulsory

[87]. The patient should be evaluated either by history or with a validated instrument such as PE profile (PEP), the PE diagnostic tool, or the index of PE if the patient has concomitant erectile dysfunction [42,88]. Imaging or laboratory studies are rarely needed, but are occasionally suggested, depending on the patient's medical history (e.g., if there is suspicion of prostatitis, a chronic pelvic pain syndrome, or hyperthyroidism) and associated ED.

7.4.5 Treatment: Nonsurgical Techniques for Sperm Retrieval

7.4.5.1 Behavioral-Psychosexual Counseling

Mostly, the couple may achieve an accommodation of the problem by using various strategies – young men with a short refractory period may oftentimes go through a second and more possessed ejaculation during a subsequent episode of intimacy. However, PE can lead to significant relationship problems for partners, such as an unhealthy sex life and generating a pattern of sexual avoidance. Importantly, this only aggravates the severity of prematurity on the occasions when intercourse does occur. The foundations of behavioral treatment are Seman's "stop–start" maneuver and its alteration proposed by Masters and Johnson, the squeeze technique. Both remedies are based on the theory that PE takes place because the man does not pay sufficient attention to pre-orgasmic levels of sexual tension [89,90]. As most men with PE are mindful of their anxiety, the sources of such anxiety being comparatively superficial, treatment success with these behavioral plans is relatively beneficial in the short term, though convincing long-term treatment effect data are absent [91–93].

7.4.5.2 Medical

Over the last two decades, an increasing number of studies have reported pharmacological treatment of PE with different medications, which act locally or centrally to delay the psychoneurological control of subsequent orgasm and ejaculation [94]. It is well demonstrated that major SSRIs and tranquilizers such as fluoxetine, paroxetine, sertraline, bupropion, clomipramine, chlorpromazine, and haloperidol delay ejaculation significantly and will result in AE in around 33 percent of men [95,96]. The efficacy of SSRIs in retarding ejaculation combined with their low side effect profile establish them as the first-line

therapeutics for PE administered either on an "on-demand" or a daily basis [97,98]. Clomipramine 10–50 mg, fluoxetine 20–40 mg, sertraline 50–100 mg, and paroxetine 20–40 mg can be used for daily treatment. Paroxetine seems to exert the strongest ejaculation delay, increasing intra-vaginal ejaculatory latency time (IELT) ~8.8 fold over baseline [99]. A recent study has reported the effects of a metered-dose aerosol spray containing a eutectic mixture of prilocaine and lidocaine. A eutectic mixture is a homogeneous mixture of two drugs that melts at a single temperature that is lower than the melting point of either of the drugs. Hence, both local anesthetics can subsist as a liquid oil rather than as crystals. The authors reported that this mixture produced a 2.4-fold increase in baseline IELT and significant improvements in the sexual quality-of-life of both patients and their partners, and also improved ejaculatory control [100]. Medications that block the phosphodiesterase type-5 isoenzyme (PDE-5), such as vardenafil, sildenafil, and tadalafil, are effective treatments for ED. Several reports have demonstrated their experience with PDE-5 inhibitors in combination with SSRIs or alone as a treatment for PE [101, 102].

7.4.5.3 Surgical Techniques

Several authors have reported the use of surgically induced penile hypoanesthesia to treat PE via hyaluronic acid gel glans penis augmentation or selective dorsal nerve neurotomy for lifelong PE refractory to pharmacological and/or behavioral treatment [103]. The role of surgery in the management of PE remains unclear, with no strong evidence supporting such modalities. Surgical techniques for sperm retrieval are not generally indicated in men with PE.

7.5 Conclusions

There are established treatment modalities for the male factor infertility attributed to sexual dysfunction such as EjD, including nonsurgical approaches in the form of medications and SSR techniques. Several sperm retrieval techniques are available, such as TESA, TESE, and MESA, in addition to PVS and EEJ. Although many hospital settings use a single technique for sperm retrieval in almost all patients, the ideal approach is personalizing the technique to each patient's clinical condition to achieve the best possible outcome.

References

1. Rosen RC. Prevalence and risk factors of sexual dysfunction in men and women. *Curr Psychiatr Rep* 2000;2:189–195.

2. Porst H, Montorsi F, Rosen RC, et al. The Premature Ejaculation Prevalence and Attitudes (PEPA) Survey: prevalence, comorbidities, and professional help-seeking. *Eur Urol* 2007;51:816–824.

3. Rowland D, McMahon CG, Abdo C, et al. Disorders of orgasm and ejaculation in men. *J Sex Med* 2010;7:1668–1686.

4. McMahon CG, Abdo C, Incrocci L, et al. Disorders of orgasm and ejaculation in men. *J Sex Med* 2004;1:58–65.

5. Hellstrom WJ. Current and future pharmacotherapies of premature ejaculation. *J Sex Med* 2006;3 (Suppl. 4):332–341

6. Bettocchi C, Verze P, Palumbo F, Arcaniolo D, Mirone V. Ejaculatory disorders: pathophysiology and management. *Nat Clin Pract Urol* 2008;5:93–103.

7. Giuliano F, Clement P. Physiology of ejaculation: emphasis on serotonergic control. *Eur Urol* 2005;48:408–417.

8. Pompeiano M, Palacios JM, Mengod G. Distribution of the serotonin 5-HT2 receptor family mRNAs: comparison between 5-HT2A and 5-HT2C receptors. *Brain Res Mol Brain Res* 1994;23:163–178.

9. Bitran D, Hull EM. Pharmacological analysis of male rat sexual behavior. *Neurosci Biobehav Rev* 1987;11:365–389.

10. Pandey SC, Davis JM, Pandey GN. Phosphoinositide system-linked serotonin receptor subtypes and their pharmacological properties and clinical correlates. *J Psychiatr Neurosci* 1995;20:215–225.

11. Giuliano F, Clement P. Serotonin and premature ejaculation: from physiology to patient management. *Eur Urol* 2006;50:454–466.

12. Cantor JM, Binik YM, Pfaus JG. Chronic fluoxetine inhibits sexual behavior in the male rat: reversal with oxytocin. *Psychopharmacology* 1999;144:355–362.

13. Roberts M, Jarvi K. Steps in the investigation and management of low semen volume in the infertile man. *Can Urol Assoc J* 2009;3:479–485.

14. Cooper TG, Noonan E, von Eckardstein S, et al. World Health Organization reference values for human semen characteristics. *Hum Reprod Update* 2010;16:231–245.

15. Kamischke A, Nieschlag E. Treatment of retrograde ejaculation and anejaculation. *Hum Reprod Update* 1999;5:448–474.

16. Ohl DA, Quallich SA, Sonksen J, Brackett NL, Lynne CM. Anejaculation and retrograde ejaculation. *Urologic Clin North Am* 2008;35:211–220.

17. Dean RC, Lue TF. Physiology of penile erection and pathophysiology of erectile dysfunction. *Urologic Clin North Am* 2005;32:379–395.

18. Everaert K, de Waard WI, Van Hoof T, et al. Neuroanatomy and neurophysiology related to sexual dysfunction in male neurogenic patients with lesions to the spinal cord or peripheral nerves. *Spinal Cord* 2010;48:182–191.

19. Dunsmuir WD, Holmes SA. The aetiology and management of erectile, ejaculatory, and fertility problems in men with diabetes mellitus. *Diabetic Med* 1996;13:700–708.

20. Rassweiler J, Teber D, Kuntz R, Hofmann R. Complications of transurethral resection of the prostate (TURP): incidence, management, and prevention. *Eur Urol* 2006;50:969–979.

21. Hisasue S, Furuya R, Itoh N, et al. Ejaculatory disorder caused by alpha-1 adrenoceptor antagonists is not retrograde ejaculation but a loss of seminal emission. *Int J Urol* 2006;13:1311–1316.

22. Rosen R, Altwein J, Boyle P, et al. Lower urinary tract symptoms and male sexual dysfunction: the multinational survey of the aging male (MSAM-7). *Eur Urol* 2003;44:637–649.

23. Vernon M, Wilson E, Muse K, Estes S, Curry T. Successful pregnancies from men with retrograde ejaculation with the use of washed sperm and gamete intrafallopian tube transfer (GIFT). *Fertil Steril* 1988;50:822–824.

24. Yavetz H, Yogev L, Hauser R, et al. Retrograde ejaculation. *Hum Reprod* 1994;9:381–386.

25. Patrick DL, Althof SE, Pryor JL, et al. Premature ejaculation: an observational study of men and their partners. *J Sex Med* 2005;2:358–367.

26. Chen J. The pathophysiology of delayed ejaculation. *Transl Androl Urol* 2016;5:549–562.

27. Jannini EA, Lenzi A. Ejaculatory disorders: epidemiology and current approaches to definition, classification and subtyping. *World J Urol* 2005;23:68–75.

28. Perelman MA, Rowland DL. Retarded ejaculation. *World J Urol* 2006;24:645–652.

29. Waldinger MD, Berendsen HH, Blok BF, Olivier B, Holstege G. Premature ejaculation and serotonergic antidepressants-induced delayed ejaculation: the involvement of the serotonergic system. *Behav Brain Res* 1998;92:111–118.

30. Corona G, Jannini EA, Vignozzi L, Rastrelli G, Maggi M. The hormonal control of ejaculation. *Nat Rev Urol* 2012;9:508–519.

31. Tamam Y, Tamam L, Akil E, Yasan A, Tamam B. Post-stroke sexual functioning in first stroke patients. *Eur J Neurol* 2008;15:660–666.

32. Corona G, Jannini EA, Mannucci E, et al. Different testosterone levels are associated with ejaculatory dysfunction. *J Sex Med* 2008;5:1991–1998.

33. Hatzimouratidis K, Amar E, Eardley I, et al. Guidelines on male sexual dysfunction: erectile dysfunction and premature ejaculation. *Eur Urol* 2010;57:804–814.

34. Sadowski DJ, Butcher MJ, Kohler TS. A review of pathophysiology and management options for delayed ejaculation. *Sex Med Rev* 2016;4:167–176.

35. Corona G, Ricca V, Bandini E, et al. Selective serotonin reuptake inhibitor-induced sexual dysfunction. *J Sex Med* 2009;6:1259–1269.

36. Stevenson JM, Bishop JR. Genetic determinants of selective serotonin reuptake inhibitor related sexual dysfunction. *Pharmacogenomics* 2014;15:1791–1806.

37. Edwards AE, Husted JR. Penile sensitivity, age, and sexual behavior. *J Clin Psychol* 1976;32:697–700.

38. Tammaro A, Parisella FR, Cavallotti C, Persechino S, Cavallotti C. Ultrastructural age-related changes in the sensory corpuscles of the human genital skin. *J Biol Reg Homeos Ag* 2013;27:241–245.

39. Rowland DL. Penile sensitivity in men: a composite of recent findings. *Urology* 1998;52:1101–1105.

40. Rowland DL, Greenleaf W, Mas M, Myers L, Davidson JM. Penile and finger sensory thresholds in young, aging, and diabetic males. *Arch Sex Behav* 1989;18:1–12.

41. Murphy JB, Lipshultz LI. Abnormalities of ejaculation. *Urol Clin North Am* 1987;14:583–596.

42. Althof SE. Sexual therapy in the age of pharmacotherapy. *Ann Rev Sex Res* 2006;17:116–131.

43. Kacker R, Morgentaler A, Pharmacotherapy for delayed orgasm after treatment for testosterone deficiency. The New England Section of American Urological Association, 83rd Annual Meeting 2014.

44. Dording CM, Mischoulon D, Petersen TJ, et al. The pharmacologic management of SSRI-induced side effects: a survey of psychiatrists. *Ann Clin Psychiatr* 2002;14:143–147.

45. Brindley GS. Electroejaculation: its technique, neurological implications and uses. *J Neurol Neurosurg Psychiatr* 1981;44:9–18.

46. Brackett NL. Semen retrieval by penile vibratory stimulation in men with spinal cord injury. *Hum Reprod Update* 1999;5:216–222.

47. Jefferys A, Siassakos D, Wardle P. The management of retrograde ejaculation: a systematic review and update. *Fertil Steril* 2012;97:306–312.

48. Ohl DA, Menge AC, Sonksen J. Penile vibratory stimulation in spinal cord injured men: optimized vibration parameters and prognostic factors. *Arch Phys Med Rehab* 1996;77:903–905.

49. Sonksen J, Biering-Sorensen F, Kristensen JK. Ejaculation induced by penile vibratory stimulation in men with spinal cord injuries: the importance of the vibratory amplitude. *Paraplegia* 1994;32:651–660.

50. Garg T, LaRosa C, Strawn E, Robb P, Sandlow JI. Outcomes after testicular aspiration and testicular tissue cryopreservation for obstructive azoospermia and ejaculatory dysfunction. *J Urol* 2008;180:2577–2580.

51. Iwahata T, Shin T, Shimomura Y, et al. Testicular sperm extraction for patients with spinal cord injury-related anejaculation: a single-center experience. *Int J Urol* 2016;23:1024–1027.

52. Yeates W. Ejaculatory disturbances. In Pryor J, Lipschultz L (eds.) *Andrology*. Butterworth, London, 1987, pp. 183–216.

53. Nesbakken A, Nygaard K, Bull-Njaa T, Carlsen E, Eri LM. Bladder and sexual dysfunction after mesorectal excision for rectal cancer. *Br J Surg* 2000;87:206–210.

54. Tiusanen H, Seitsalo S, Osterman K, Soini J. Retrograde ejaculation after anterior interbody lumbar fusion. *Eur Spine J* 1995;4:339–342.

55. Donohue JP, Foster RS. Retroperitoneal lymphadenectomy in staging and treatment: the development of nerve-sparing techniques. *Urol Clin North Am* 1998;25:461–468.

56. Gessa GL, Tagliamonte A. Role of brain monoamines in male sexual behavior. *Life Sci* 1974;14:425–436.

57. Clement P, Bernabe J, Kia HK, Alexandre L, Giuliano F. D2-like receptors mediate the expulsion phase of ejaculation elicited by 8-hydroxy-2-(di-N-propylamino) tetralin in rats. *J Pharmacol Exp Ther* 2006;316:830–834.

58. Sabanegh E Jr., Agarwal A. Male infertility. In: Wein AJ, Kavoussi LR, Novick A, Partin AW, Peters CA (ed.) *Cambell-Walsh Urology*. Saunders, Philadelphia, PA, 2012, pp. 616–647.

59. van der Linden PJ, Nan PM, te Velde ER, van Kooy RJ. Retrograde ejaculation: successful treatment with artificial insemination. *Obstet Gynecol* 1992;79:126–128.

60. Shoshany O, Abhyankar N, Elyaguov J, Niederberger C. Efficacy of treatment with

pseudoephedrine in men with retrograde ejaculation. *Andrology* 2017;5:744–748.

61. Ochsenkuhn R, Kamischke A, Nieschlag E. Imipramine for successful treatment of retrograde ejaculation caused by retroperitoneal surgery. *Int J Androl* 1999;22:173–177.

62. Braude PR, Ross LD, Bolton VN, Ockenden K. Retrograde ejaculation: a systematic approach to non-invasive recovery of spermatozoa from post-ejaculatory urine for artificial insemination. *Br J Obstet Gynecol* 1987;94:76–83.

63. Reynolds JC, McCall A, Kim ED, Lipshultz LI. Bladder neck collagen injection restores antegrade ejaculation after bladder neck surgery. *J Urol* 1998;159:1303.

64. Dees JE. Congenital epispadias with incontinence. *J Urol* 1949;62:513–522.

65. Abrahams JI, Solish GI, Boorjian P, Waterhouse RK. The surgical correction of retrograde ejaculation. *J Urol* 1975;114:888–890.

66. Lochner-Ernst D, Mandalka B, Kramer G, Stohrer M. Conservative and surgical semen retrieval in patients with spinal cord injury. *Spinal Cord* 1997;35:463–468.

67. Wagenknecht LV, Weitze KH, Hoppe LP, et al. Microsurgery in andrologic urology: II. Alloplastic spermatocele. *J Microsurg* 1980;1:428–435.

68. Wagenknecht LV, Weitze KH, Hoppe LP, et al. New development in surgical andrology: alloplastic spermatocele. *Investigat Urol* 1980;17:432–434.

69. Brindley GS, Scott GI, Hendry WF. Vas cannulation with implanted sperm reservoirs for obstructive azoospermia or ejaculatory failure. *Br J Urol* 1986;58:721–723.

70. Berger RE, Muller CH, Smith D, et al. Operative recovery of vasal sperm from anejaculatory men: preliminary report. *J Urol* 1986;135:948–950.

71. Rosenlund B, Sjoblom P, Tornblom M, Hultling C, Hillensjo T. In-vitro fertilization and intracytoplasmic sperm injection in the treatment of infertility after testicular cancer. *Hum Reprod* 1998;13:414–418.

72. Middleton RG, Urry RL. The Young–Dees operation for the correction of retrograde ejaculation. *J Urol* 1986;136:1208–1209.

73. Serefoglu EC, McMahon CG, Waldinger MD, et al. An evidence-based unified definition of lifelong and acquired premature ejaculation: report of the Second International Society for Sexual Medicine Ad Hoc Committee for the Definition of Premature Ejaculation. *J Sex Med* 2014;11:1423–1441.

74. Althof SE, McMahon CG, Waldinger MD, et al. An update of the International Society of Sexual Medicine's guidelines for the diagnosis and treatment of premature ejaculation (PE). *Sex Med* 2014;2:60–90.

75. Corona G, Petrone L, Mannucci E, et al. Psycho-biological correlates of rapid ejaculation in patients attending an andrologic unit for sexual dysfunctions. *Eur Urol* 2004;46:615–622.

76. Lawall C, Ezeh U, Turek PJ. How semen quality changes in hypogonadal men on clomiphene citrate. *Fertil Steril* 2004;82:S21.

77. Laumann EO, Paik A, Rosen RC. Sexual dysfunction in the United States: prevalence and predictors. *JAMA* 1999;281:537–544.

78. Reading AE, Wiest WM. An analysis of self-reported sexual behavior in a sample of normal males. *Arch Sex Behav* 1984;13:69–83.

79. Spector KR, Boyle M. The prevalence and perceived aetiology of male sexual problems in a non-clinical sample. *Br J Med Psychol* 1986;59(Pt 4):351–358.

80. Basile Fasolo C, Mirone V, Gentile V, et al. Premature ejaculation: prevalence and associated conditions in a sample of 12,558 men attending the andrology prevention week 2001–2014: a study of the Italian Society of Andrology (SIA). *J Sex Med* 2005;2:376–382.

81. Tignol J, Martin-Guehl C, Aouizerate B, Grabot D, Auriacombe M. Social phobia and premature ejaculation: a case–control study. *Depress Anxiety* 2006;23:153–157.

82. Kaplan HS, Kohl RN, Pomeroy WB, Offit AK, Hogan B. Group treatment of premature ejaculation. *Arch Sex Behav* 1974;3:443–452.

83. Schapiro B. Premature ejaculation: a review of 1130 cases. *J Urol* 1943;50:374–379.

84. Waldinger MD. The neurobiological approach to premature ejaculation. *J Urol* 2002;168:2359–2367.

85. Waldinger MD, Hengeveld MW, Zwinderman AH, Olivier B. Effect of SSRI antidepressants on ejaculation: a double-blind, randomized, placebo-controlled study with fluoxetine, fluvoxamine, paroxetine, and sertraline. *J Clin Psychopharmacol* 1998;18:274–281.

86. Vandereycken W. Towards a better delineation of ejaculatory disorders. *Acta Psychiatrica Belgica* 1986;86:57–63.

87. Althof SE, McMahon CG, Waldinger MD, et al. An update of the International Society of Sexual Medicine's guidelines for the diagnosis and treatment of premature ejaculation (PE). *J Sex Med* 2014;11:1392–1422.

88. Patrick DL, Giuliano F, Ho KF, et al. The premature ejaculation profile: validation of self-reported outcome measures for research and practice. *BJU Int* 2009;103:358–364.

89. Masters WH JV. *Human Sexual Inadequacy*. Little, Brown, Boston, MA, 1970.

90. Semans JH. Premature ejaculation: a new approach. *South Med J* 1956;49:353–358.

91. De Amicis LA, Goldberg DC, LoPiccolo J, Friedman J, Davies L. Clinical follow-up of couples treated for sexual dysfunction. *Arch Sex Behav* 1985;14:467–489.

92. de Carufel F, Trudel G. Effects of a new functional-sexological treatment for premature ejaculation. *J Sex Marital Ther* 2006;32:97–114.

93. Hawton K, Catalan J, Martin P, Fagg J. Long-term outcome of sex therapy. *Behav Res Ther* 1986;24:665–675.

94. Montague DK, Jarow J, Broderick GA, et al. AUA guideline on the pharmacologic management of premature ejaculation. *J Urol* 2004;172:290–294.

95. DeVeaugh-Geiss J, Landau P, Katz R. Preliminary results from a multicenter trial of clomipramine in obsessive-compulsive disorder. *Psychopharmacol Bull* 1989;25:36–40.

96. Kotin J, Wilbert DE, Verburg D, Soldinger SM. Thioridazine and sexual dysfunction. *Am J Psychiatr* 1976;133:82–85.

97. McMahon CG, Touma K. Treatment of premature ejaculation with paroxetine hydrochloride as needed: 2 single-blind placebo controlled crossover studies. *J Urol* 1999;161:1826–1830.

98. Waldinger MD, Berendsen HHG, Blok BFM, Olivier B, Holstege G. Premature ejaculation and serotonergic antidepressants-induced delayed ejaculation: the involvement of the serotonergic system. *Behav Brain Res* 1998;92:111–118.

99. Waldinger MD. Towards evidence-based drug treatment research on premature ejaculation: a critical evaluation of methodology. *Int J Impot Res* 2003;15:309–313.

100. Dinsmore WW, Hackett G, Goldmeier D, et al. Topical eutectic mixture for premature ejaculation (TEMPE): a novel aerosol-delivery form of lidocaine–prilocaine for treating premature ejaculation. *BJU Int* 2007;99:369–375.

101. Abdel-Hamid IA, El Naggar EA, El Gilany AH. Assessment of as needed use of pharmacotherapy and the pause-squeeze technique in premature ejaculation. *Int J Impot Res* 2001;13:41–45.

102. Salonia A, Maga T, Colombo R, et al. A prospective study comparing paroxetine alone versus paroxetine plus sildenafil in patients with premature ejaculation. *J Urol* 2002;168:2486–2489.

103. Kim JJ, Kwak TI, Jeon BG, Cheon J, Moon DG. Effects of glans penis augmentation using hyaluronic acid gel for premature ejaculation. *Int J Impot Res* 2004;16:547–551.

Sperm Retrieval in Non-azoospermic Men
Indications, Protocol, and Outcomes

Sandro C. Esteves and Ahmad Majzoub

8.1 Introduction

The development of intracytoplasmic sperm injection (ICSI) was an extraordinary achievement in the field of assisted reproduction technology (ART) [1]. The method was initially introduced in 1992 as a modification of conventional *in vitro* fertilization (IVF), enabling men with low sperm quantity and quality to father a biological child [2]. Nowadays, ICSI has become the most commonly used method of fertilization in ART, and it is the method of choice for overcoming untreatable severe male factor infertility [3].

8.1.1 Sperm Retrieval in Azoospermic Men

A few years after the introduction of ICSI, methods to harvest sperm from the epididymides and testes were developed to help men with azoospermia overcome infertility (reviewed in [4]). Azoospermia is a condition that affects approximately 10–15 percent of men with infertility and is characterized by a complete absence of spermatozoa in the ejaculate [5]. Before ICSI, few options were available for the affected men to father a biological child, in particular, for those with nonobstructive azoospermia [6]. The latter is associated with untreatable testicular disorders that result in spermatogenic failure. Nevertheless, 30–60 percent of men with nonobstructive azoospermia have focal testicular sperm production that can be retrieved and used for ICSI [7]. By contrast, obstructive azoospermia results from bilateral obstruction of the seminal ducts. Spermatogenesis is intact in men with obstructive azoospermia; therefore, sperm can be retrieved from epididymides or testicles in virtually all cases [8].

Nowadays, the two methods most commonly used to harvest sperm in men with azoospermia are percutaneous acquisition and open surgery (with or without the aid of microsurgery) [9]. In men with obstructive azoospermia, the sperm retrieval technique and the cause of obstructive azoospermia have little impact on sperm retrieval success and ICSI outcome [8]. Among men with nonobstructive azoospermia, the use of microsurgical TESE (testicular sperm extraction) yields higher sperm retrieval success rates and fewer complications than conventional TESE (reviewed in [7]). After retrieval of epididymal or testicular sperm, ICSI is used instead of conventional IVF as the retrieved gametes are unable to fertilize the oocytes by conventional IVF.

8.1.2 Sperm Retrieval in Non-azoospermic Men

Ejaculated sperm are generally regarded as having the highest fertilization potential as they have completed their transit through the male reproductive tract. Furthermore, the early ICSI experience suggested that sperm parameters – evaluated on ejaculated semen; namely, concentration, motility, and morphology – had no significant influence on outcomes [10]. However, as experience accumulated, reports of an association between sperm quality and ICSI outcomes increased steadily [11–13]. Concerns of a possible role of the paternal gamete on poor ICSI outcomes have been raised, in particular, in cases where (1) ejaculated specimens containing abnormal levels of sperm with damaged chromatin were used for sperm injections; and (2) the number (and quality) of ejaculated sperm was too low (e.g., cryptozoospermia, which is denoted by absence or very few spermatozoa in the fresh ejaculate but observed after microscopic examination of centrifuged pellet).

8.1.2.1 Biological Plausibility

It is well-established that sperm chromatin integrity is vital for the birth of healthy infants [14]. In ART, fertilization of oocytes by sperm with damaged chromatin might lead to an increased risk of fertilization failure, embryo development arrest, implantation failure, miscarriage, congenital malformations, as well as perinatal and postnatal morbidity [15–17]. The causes of sperm chromatin damage include apoptosis during spermatogenesis, deficient chromatin remodeling during spermiogenesis [18], activation of endogenous caspases and endonucleases [19], exogenous factors such as environmental toxicants, radiotherapy, and chemotherapy [20], and oxidative stress [21]. In normal conditions, there is an equilibrium between reactive oxygen species (ROS) production and antioxidant defense system in the male reproductive tract. When ROS production overwhelms antioxidant defenses, a state of oxidative stress ensues. As a result, excessive ROS attack both sperm membranes and nuclear and mitochondrial DNA, mostly during sperm transit through the male reproductive tract [20–22].

Non-azoospermic infertile men often have high levels of sperm chromatin damage in their neat semen [23,24]. Abnormal levels of sperm chromatin damage have been demonstrated primarily in ejaculates of men with poor conventional semen parameters (count, motility, morphology), although counterparts with semen analysis within normal ranges might also be affected [25,26]. Varicocele, systemic diseases, male accessory gland infections, advanced paternal age, obesity, lifestyle and environmental factors, radiation, and heat exposure are some of the conditions associated with sperm chromatin damage (reviewed in [27]). Most of these stressors share oxidative stress as a common trait.

However, data from human studies indicate that sperm chromatin damage is lower in testicular sperm than in epididymal and ejaculated sperm. This evidence derives from studies involving men with obstructive azoospermia as well as non-azoospermic counterparts, as discussed below.

In a study involving men with obstructive azoospermia, Steele et al. observed that the frequency of sperm with intact chromatin – assessed by the Comet assay – in paired samples of testicular and epididymal spermatozoa was higher in the former (83.0 ± 1.2 percent versus 75.4 ± 2.3 percent, $p < 0.05$). [28]. In a similar study involving 25 men with obstructive azoospermia, O'Connell et al. showed the testicular sperm had better quality than epididymal sperm [29]. The authors used polymerase chain reaction (PCR) and alkaline Comet assay to assess mitochondrial DNA (mtDNA) and nuclear DNA (nDNA), respectively. Testicular sperm had significantly more wild-type mtDNA and lower incidence of multiple deletions and smaller mtDNA fragments than epididymal sperm, whereas epididymal sperm displayed more

large-scale deletions ($p < 0.05$). In their study, a strong correlation was found between nuclear DNA damage, the number of mtDNA deletions ($r = 0.48$, $r = 0.50$, $p < 0.0001$) and deletion size ($r = 0.58$, $r = 0.60$, $p < 0.001$) in both epididymal and testicular sperm. Lastly, Hammoud et al., using the terminal deoxynucleotidyl transferase-mediated dUTP-biotin nick-end labeling (TUNEL) assay, assessed the levels of sperm chromatin damage in paired testicular and epididymal specimens of 21 men with obstructive azoospermia [30]. Sperm chromatin damage values were lower in the testis (6.7 ± 0.7 percent) than in the epididymis (caput: 14.9 ± 1.9 percent; $p = 0.0007$; and corpus/cauda: 32.6 ± 3.1 percent; $p < 0.0001$).

Likewise, studies assessing paired testicular and ejaculated specimens of non-azoospermic men demonstrate better chromatin integrity in the former. In 2005, Greco et al. published the first series showing that the rates of sperm exhibiting chromatin damage was lower in testicular sperm than ejaculated sperm (TUNEL assay; testis: 4.8 ± 3.6 percent [testis] versus 23.6 ± 5.1 percent [ejaculate]) [31]. Later, in 2010, Moskovtsev et al. confirmed these findings in a group of men with persistent high sperm chromatin damage in neat semen after use of oral antioxidants (TUNEL assay: 13.3 ± 7.3 percent [testis] versus 39.7 ± 14.8 percent [ejaculate], $p < 0.001$) [32]. Another cohort study by the same authors published in 2012 showed similar results (TUNEL assay: 14.9 percent [testis] versus 40.6 percent [ejaculate]) [33]. In 2015, Esteves et al. used the sperm chromatin dispersion (SCD) assay to evaluate paired testicular and ejaculated specimens of a large cohort of men with idiopathic oligozoospermia and high rates of sperm chromatin damage on neat ejaculate [34]. In their study, testicular sperm had fivefold lower rates of sperm chromatin damage than ejaculated sperm (8.3 ± 5.3 percent versus 40.7 ± 9.9 percent, respectively; $p < 0.001$). In another 2015 cohort study of men with severe oligozoospermia, Mehta et al. also showed less chromatin damage in testicular sperm compared to ejaculated sperm (TUNEL assay: 5 percent versus 24 percent, respectively; $p < 0.001$) [35]. A 2017 systematic review – followed by meta-analysis – compiled the results of these five studies [36] and showed that the mean difference (MD) in sperm DNA fragmentation rates – a measure of sperm chromatin damage – was −24.6 percent (95 percent CI –32.5 to –16.6; $I^2 = 92$ percent; $p < 0.001$). Four studies used the TUNEL assay for the assessment of SDF (pooled MD:

−19.8 percent; 95 percent CI −22.3 to −17.2; $I^2 = 15$ percent; $p < 0.001$), whereas one study used the SCD assay (MD: −32.4 percent; 95 percent CI −34.85 to −29.95; $p < 0.001$).

In conclusion, fair evidence indicates that among infertile men, sperm chromatin integrity progressively decreases as sperm transit across the genital tract. The mechanisms are not fully understood, but apparently, oxidative attack after sperm release from the seminiferous tubules is the main reason for the higher frequency of sperm with damaged chromatin in both epididymal and ejaculated sperm than testicular sperm. These findings, combined with the observations of possible improved ICSI outcomes with the use of sperm retrieved from the testes in preference

over ejaculated sperm – discussed in the next sections – have led to the extended indications of sperm retrieval.

8.2 Indications

Table 8.1 lists the indications for sperm retrieval in non-azoospermic infertile males.

8.3 Protocol

Both percutaneous and open sperm retrieval procedures can be used to harvest sperm from the seminiferous tubules in non-azoospermic men. These methods are commonly carried out on an outpatient basis and the same day as oocyte retrieval.

Table 8.1 Extended indications of sperm retrieval for non-azoospermic infertile men

Type of male infertility	Fertilization method	Level of evidence	References	Grade of recommendation
Elevated levels of sperm with chromatin damage on neat ejaculate§	ICSI mandatory	2a 2b 4	36 34, 37–40 19, 30, 34, 41	B–C
Severe oligozoospermia and cryptozoospermia*	ICSI mandatory	2b 3a 3b 4	42–44 45, 46 47–49 50	B–C

ICSI, intracytoplasmic sperm injection.

§ Assessed by the four most common assays, namely TUNEL, SCD, Comet, and sperm chromatin structure assay (SCSA); in this scenario, testicular sperm retrieval could be offered as a means to improve ICSI outcomes, in particular for men with persistent high levels of sperm with damaged chromatin on the neat ejaculate – despite all efforts to treat any cause associated with sperm chromatin damage.

*No or extremely rare spermatozoa in the fresh ejaculate but observed after microscopic examination of centrifuged pellet.

Level 2a: systematic review with homogeneity of cohort studies; homogeneity defined by lack of worrisome variations (heterogeneity) in the directions and degrees of results between individual studies.

Level 2b: Individual cohort study (including low-quality randomized controlled trials [RCT]).

Level 3a: Systematic review with homogeneity of case–control studies; homogeneity defined by lack of worrisome variations (heterogeneity) in the directions and degrees of results between individual studies.

Level 3b: Individual case–control study.

Level 4: Case series and poor-quality cohort and case–control studies. Poor-quality cohort studies denoted by those that failed to clearly define comparison groups and/or failed to measure exposures and outcomes in the same (preferably blinded), objective way in both exposed and non-exposed individuals and/or failed to identify or appropriately control known confounders and/or failed to carry out a sufficiently long and complete follow-up of patients. Poor-quality case–control studies denoted by those that failed to clearly define comparison groups and/or failed to measure exposures and outcomes in the same (preferably blinded), objective way in both cases and controls and/or failed to identify or appropriately control known confounders.

Grade B: consistent level 2 or 3 studies or extrapolations from level 1 studies (systematic reviews with homogeneity of RCT and individual RCT with narrow confidence interval).

Grade C: level 4 studies or extrapolations from level 2 or 3 studies. Extrapolations are where data is used in a situation that has potentially clinically important differences to the original study situation.

Grade D: level 5 evidence (denoted by expert opinion without explicit critical appraisal, or studies based on physiology, bench research or "first principles") or troublingly inconsistent or inconclusive studies of any level.

Levels of evidence and grades of recommendation according to 'Oxford Centre for Evidence-based Medicine – Levels of Evidence (March 2009)', available at: www.cebm.net/2009/06/oxford-centre-evidence-based-medicine-levels-evidence-march-2009.

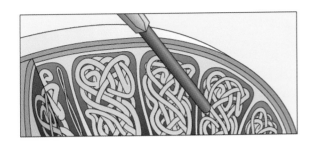

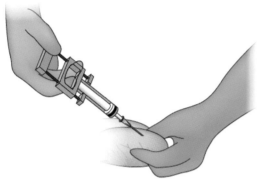

Figure 8.1 Testicular sperm aspiration. A 18 G needle connected to a 20 ml syringe fit to the Cameco holder is percutaneously inserted into the testis. Negative pressure is created, and the tip of the needle is moved within the testis to disrupt the seminiferous tubules and sample different areas. Adapted by permission from Macmillan Publishers Ltd: Nature Reviews Urology. Esteves SC, Roque M, Bedoschi G, Haahr T, Humaidan P. Intracytoplasmic sperm injection for male infertility and consequences for offspring, issue 15, pages 535–562, 2018

8.3.1 Percutaneous

8.3.1.1 Testicular Sperm Aspiration

Testicular sperm aspiration (TESA) is carried out under local anesthesia applied to the spermatic cord, intravenous sedation or general anesthesia (Figure 8.1) [4]. The testicle is held firmly and punctured using a large gauge needle (e.g., 18 G) attached to a syringe. The needle is introduced at an oblique angle in its anterior aspect of the upper pole to decrease the risk of vascular injury. Loupe magnification may be used during puncture to avoid transfixing scrotal vessels seen through the skin [6]. Negative pressure is applied using different maneuvers (e.g., Cameco syringe holder; Figure 8.1) to aid extraction of seminiferous tubules. The seminiferous tubules are disrupted by moving the needle back and forth so they can be easily aspirated. The sample is immediately analyzed in the IVF laboratory and, if adequate, the procedure is finished; otherwise, the contralateral testis is punctured at the same operative time. A short movie depicting the main steps

of the procedure can be found at www.youtube.com/watch?v=o9MgknYEzN0.

8.3.2 Open Non-microsurgical

8.3.2.1 Testicular Sperm Extraction

Testicular sperm extraction is carried under local anesthesia, intravenous sedation combined with local anesthesia, spinal block, or general anesthesia [6]. The procedure can be performed with or without testis delivery. The skin and subjacent layers are incised transversally to expose the tunica albuginea, which is opened with a sharp knife. Typically, a small transversal albuginea opening (0.5–1.0 cm incision) is made at the mid-testicular pole, and one or multiple fragments of the parenchyma is cut off with the aid of scissors or forceps [51] (Figure 8.2). The tunica albuginea is closed with either non-absorbable or absorbable sutures, whereas the tunica vaginalis, dartos, and skin are sutured with absorbable suture.

8.3.3 Open Microsurgical

8.3.3.1 Microdissection Testicular Sperm Extraction

Microdissection testicular sperm extraction (micro-TESE) – initially described by Schlegel in 1996 – can be performed under intravenous sedation combined with local anesthesia, general anesthesia or spinal block [6,51,52]. After skin incision, the testis is delivered outside the scrotum. The tunica albuginea is widely incised transversally, and the testicular parenchyma is exposed (Figure 8.3). The operating microscope with optical magnification ranging of 16–25× is used, and dissection of seminiferous tubules is carried out in search of enlarged tubules that are more likely to contain mature sperm. During dissection, damage to the intratesticular blood supply is actively avoided. Extracted specimens are transferred to the IVF laboratory for examination. A short movie depicting the main steps of the procedure can be found at www.brazjurol.com.br/videos/may_june_2013/Esteves_440_441video.htm [53].

8.3.4 Laboratory Sperm Handling

Methods to remove cellular debris and red blood cells are generally used to prepare the extracted specimens for ICSI. Since iatrogenic sperm DNA damage can occur during sperm processing, all efforts should be made to minimize such damage. Controlling centrifugation force and duration, limiting exposure to ultraviolet light and temperature variation, optimizing

59

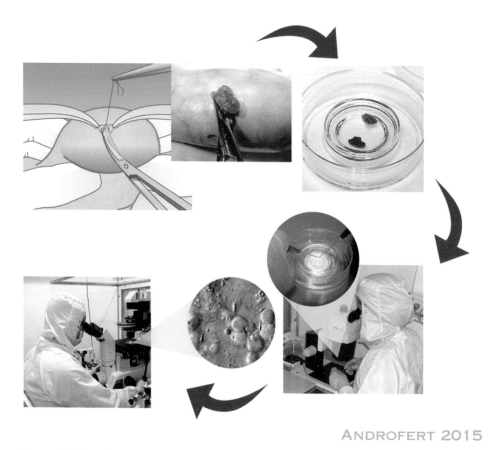

Figure 8.2 Testicular sperm extraction (TESE). Single or multiple incisions are made on the tunica albuginea and one or several testicular biopsies are taken. Extracted specimens are placed on a Petri dish with culture media and sent to the laboratory for processing by mechanical mincing under the stereomicroscope. The cell suspension is examined under the inverted microscope for sperm search. After confirmation of an adequate number of sperm for ICSI, specimens are incubated at room temperature until sperm injections take place. Reprinted with permission, ANDROFERT. All rights reserved

laboratory air quality conditions, and using high-quality reagents, culture media, and disposable materials are critical elements [54,55]. Whenever possible, techniques aimed at improving the sperm fertilizing potential should be applied, including the use of chemical stimulants and/or methods to select viable sperm for ICSI. The latter is particularly important when only immotile spermatozoa are harvested. Table 8.2 provides an overview of the laboratory processes concerning the processing of surgically extracted specimens. A detailed laboratory procedure for processing such specimens can be found elsewhere [56].

Importantly, ICSI should be carried out immediately after completion of sperm processing. Prolonged sperm incubation, in particular, at 37 °C, and sperm freezing might negatively affect sperm chromatin damage [22,57,58]. Therefore, sperm retrieval for non-azoospermic men should be scheduled on the same day as oocyte retrieval.

8.4 Outcomes

8.4.1 Sperm Retrieval Success Rates

Sperm retrieval success rates in the context of non-azoospermic men are virtually 100 percent [36]. Such men are either oligozoospermic or normozoospermic, thus exhibiting relatively well-preserved sperm production. The seminiferous tubules of men with normozoospermia invariably contain mature sperm; therefore, both percutaneous and open testicular sperm retrieval can be used with similar success rates [59]. By contrast, men with oligozoospermia show varying degrees of sperm production and the choice of the sperm retrieval technique might play a role,

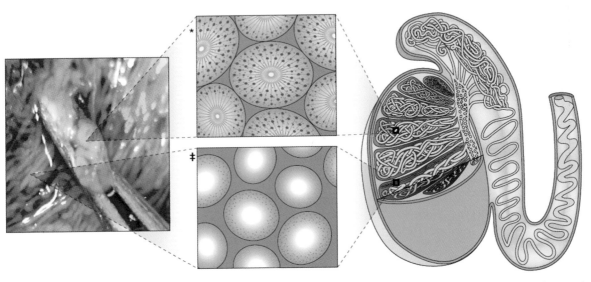

Figure 8.3 Microsurgical testicular sperm extraction. After the testicle is exteriorized, a single and large incision is made in an avascular area of the albuginea to expose the seminiferous tubules. The dilated tubules are identified and removed with micro-forceps. The illustration in the middle of the figure depicts histopathology cross-sections of a dilated seminiferous tubule with active spermatogenesis and a thin tubule with germ cell aplasia. Adapted by permission from Macmillan Publishers Ltd: Nature Reviews Urology. Esteves SC, Roque M, Bedoschi G, Haahr T, Humaidan P. Intracytoplasmic sperm injection for male infertility and consequences for offspring, issue 15, pages 535–562, 2018

particularly for men with severe oligozoospermia. While similar success rates can be achieved by percutaneous and open sperm retrieval methods in men with mild and moderate oligozoospermia [34], open methods, in particular microsurgical ones, should be preferred in men with severe oligozoospermia to increase the likelihood of harvesting sperm and decrease the risk of complications [35].

8.4.2 Sperm Retrieval Complications

Sperm retrieval complications include pain, swelling, infection, hematoma, and loss of testicular function [4,51]. The complication rates are reported to be less than 5 percent overall, most of which resolve spontaneously without compromising testicular function [51,60]. A transient decline in testosterone levels is expected after open procedures, which tend to return to preoperative values in approximately 6–12 months [60]. However, large-volume tissue extraction, mainly using non-microsurgical multiple biopsy TESE, can cause testicular damage (reviewed in [7]). Testicular atrophy and permanent reduction in androgen production have been occasionally reported after TESE, which might cause hypogonadism [61].

Nevertheless, most of the data mentioned above relate to studies involving men with azoospermia. In the context of non-azoospermic men, sperm retrieval is

associated with very few complications as minimal tissue extraction yields sufficient numbers of sperm for ICSI [62]. Yet, given the potential risk for complications and adverse effects on testicular function, sperm retrieval should be performed by well-trained urologists.

8.4.3 Pregnancy Outcomes

8.4.3.1 Sperm chromatin damage

In 2005, Greco et al. published the first successful series of ICSI using testicular sperm in 18 non-azoospermic patients with high sperm chromatin damage on neat semen [31]. On the day of oocyte retrieval, the male partners underwent TESA or TESE. In this series, intracytoplasmic testicular sperm injection resulted in eight clinical pregnancies (44.5 percent), whereas only one pregnancy (5.6 percent) that ended in miscarriage had been obtained in previous cycles.

Later in 2010, Sakkas and Alvarez reported on 72 patients with high levels of sperm chromatin damage on neat semen who used testicular sperm for ICSI [20]. Testicular sperm aspiration was used to harvest sperm from the seminiferous tubules. In this series, the clinical pregnancy rates and implantation rates were higher after ICSI using testicular sperm than ejaculated sperm (40.0 percent and 28.1 percent versus 13.8 percent and 6.5 percent, respectively; $p < 0.05$).

Table 8.2 Laboratory strategies to handle testicular specimens retrieved from non-azoospermic men

Process	Procedures	Techniques	Main goal	Critical level
Testicular tissue processing	Mechanical tissue mincing	Disruption of seminiferous tubules using fine needles or micro-scissors, and forced pass through small diameter catheters	Tubular breakdown and cellular content loss	Critical
	Red blood cell lysis	Incubation of testicular suspensions with erythrocyte lysing buffer solution	Removal of excessive blood cells from testicular specimens	Optional
	Motility enhancement	Incubation of testicular specimens with pentoxifylline	Selection of viable sperm for ICSI	Optional
Laboratory environment and laboratory practices	Air quality control	Air particulate and volatile organic compounds filtration	Secure optimal safety conditions for gamete handling, sperm injection, and embryo culture	Recommended
	Maintenance of temperature and pH stability	Quality control and quality assurance of instruments, equipment, and reagents	Avoid iatrogenic cellular damage	Critical
	Centrifugation	Simple washing with buffered medium or mini-gradient centrifugation using low centrifugation forces	Avoid iatrogenic cellular damage	Critical
	Sterile techniques	Manipulation of gametes and embryos in laminar flow cabinets or inside controlled environments	Secure optimal safety conditions for gamete handling, sperm injection, and embryo culture	Critical
Intracytoplasmic sperm injection	Sperm selection	Hypo-osmotic swelling test, mechanical touch technique, and laser-assisted sperm selection	Selection of viable immotile sperm for ICSI	Optional

In 2015, Esteves et al. reported the first prospective comparative study investigating the efficacy of use of testicular sperm for ICSI among men with idiopathic oligozoospermia and high sperm chromatin damage in neat semen [34]. On the day of oocyte retrieval, either TESA or conventional TESE were used for sperm retrieval. In this series that included 172 patients with no history of ICSI failure, the live birth rate was higher with testicular sperm (versus ejaculated sperm), with an adjusted relative risk of 1.76 (95 percent CI 1.15–2.70; $p = 0.008$). The authors reported that approximately five patients had to be treated to result in one additional live birth by testicular sperm for ICSI compared to ejaculated sperm.

Also in 2015, Mehta et al. published another successful series of ICSI using sperm retrieved from the testis of 24 patients with severe oligozoospermia and history of failed ICSI [35]. The male partners underwent micro-TESE, in which the seminiferous tubules were dissected, mature sperm were identified, and the extracted sperm were used for ICSI. In this series, 12 clinical pregnancies were achieved, all of which resulted in live births.

In a 2016 large retrospective cohort study evaluating ICSI outcomes in patients with high sperm chromatin damage on neat semen in Australia, Bradley et al. reported that ICSI with testicular sperm resulted in higher live birth rates (49.8 percent) than ICSI with ejaculated sperm, even when advanced laboratory methods – intracytoplasmic morphologically selected sperm injection (IMSI) and hyaluronic acid sperm selection ICSI (PICSI) – were used to select ejaculated sperm with better chromatin integrity for ICSI (38.3 percent and 28.7 percent, respectively; $p = 0.02$) [37].

Later in 2017, Pabuccu et al. investigated the efficacy of use of testicular sperm for ICSI among normozoospermic men and high sperm chromatin damage in neat semen [38]. Seventy-one couples with a history of ICSI failure were included. On the day of oocyte retrieval, TESA was used to harvest sperm from the seminiferous tubules. In this series, ICSI with testicular sperm was associated with higher rates of clinical pregnancy (41.9 versus 20.0 percent; $p = 0.04$) and ongoing pregnancy (38.7 versus 15.0 percent; $p = 0.02$) than with ejaculated sperm.

A systematic review published in 2017 aggregated the evidence of the studies mentioned above concerning the use of testicular sperm for ICSI in men with high sperm chromatin damage in semen. A total of 507 ICSI cycles in which 3840 oocytes were injected with either ejaculated sperm or testicular sperm was included. Using meta-analysis, the authors showed higher clinical pregnancy rate (OR 3.6, 95 percent CI 1.94–6.69; $I^2 = 0$ percent; $p < 0.0001$) and live birth rate (OR 2.6, 95 percent CI 1.54–4.35, $I^2 = 0$ percent; $p = 0.0003$), and lower miscarriage rates (OR 0.40, 95 percent CI 0.10–1.65, $I^2 = 34$ percent; $p = 0.005$) when comparing Testi-ICSI with ejaculated ICSI [36].

Subsequently, in 2018, Arafa et al. assessed ICSI outcomes with the use of testicular sperm in 36 men with high sperm chromatin damage in semen [41]. The male partners had either normozoospermia or oligozoospermia, and TESA was used for sperm retrieval. The couples reported a history of ICSI failure with use of ejaculated sperm. In this series, the rates of clinical pregnancy were higher with Testi-ICSI than ejaculated sperm ICSI (38.9 versus 13.8 percent; $p < 0.0001$). Of these pregnancies, 17 were reported to result in live offspring in the testicular sperm ICSI group compared to only three in the ejaculated sperm ICSI group.

Also in 2018, Zhang et al. compared ICSI outcomes by testicular sperm versus ejaculated sperm in a group of 102 infertile men [39]. Like the reports mentioned above, the male partners had high rates of sperm chromatin damage in neat semen. The rates of clinical pregnancy (36.0 versus 14.6 percent; $p = 0.017$) and delivery (36.0 versus 9.8 percent; $p = 0.001$) were higher after the transfer of embryos resulting from Testi-ICSI than ejaculated sperm for ICSI.

Lastly, in 2019, Herrero et al. investigated the use of Testi-ICSI in 145 couples with no previous live births and a history of at least two previous failed ICSI cycles with ejaculated sperm [40]. The studied

men had high levels of sperm chromatin damage on neat semen, and TESE was the method used to harvest sperm from the seminiferous tubules. In this series, cumulative live birth rates were higher after use of Testi-ICSI than ejaculated sperm for ICSI (21.7 versus 9.1 percent; $p < 0.01$).

Collectively, data from six retrospective studies and three prospective studies, including a total of 830 patients and 902 ICSI cycles, suggest that ICSI with testicular sperm is superior to ICSI with ejaculated sperm to overcome infertility among non-azoospermic men with high sperm chromatin damage in semen (Table 8.3). Testi-ICSI has been postulated to bypass post-testicular sperm chromatin damage caused by oxidative stress during sperm transit through the epididymis. As a result, the chances of oocyte fertilization by genomically intact testicular spermatozoa are increased, thus resulting in an increased possibility of formation of a normal embryonic genome and an increased likelihood of achieving a live birth. However, no RCT has yet investigated the efficiency of testicular sperm in non-azoospermic men with sperm chromatin damage.

8.4.3.2 Severe Oligozoospermia and Cryptozoospermia

The first successful series of ICSI with testicular sperm in patients with severe oligozoospermia was reported by Weissman et al. in 2008 [50]. The authors performed testicular sperm injections in four couples with a history of multiple failed IVF/ICSI cycles after the use of poor-quality ejaculated sperm. The male partners had sperm count ranging from 0.2 to 2.0 million/ml. On the day of oocyte retrieval, TESA was performed, and in all cases, motile spermatozoa were retrieved. Embryo implantation and delivery of healthy offspring were established after embryo transfers in all couples.

In the same year, Bendikson et al. reported the first study investigating the efficacy of Testi-ICSI in patients with cryptozoospermia [47]. The authors searched their database of nonobstructive azoospermic patients who had a few viable sperm in the ejaculate after centrifugation on the day of sperm retrieval. Sixteen patients met the inclusion criteria, and underwent 27 ejaculated and 21 testicular ICSI cycles. The fertilization rates between ejaculate and testicular groups (51.7 versus 59.9 percent, $p < 0.05$) were not different. However, the implantation rate was higher after testicular ICSI than ejaculate ICSI (20.3 versus 7.0 percent; $p < 0.05$). Fourteen

Table 8.3 Characteristics and main outcome measures of studies reporting ICSI outcomes with testicular versus ejaculated sperm in non-azoospermic men with high sperm DNA fragmentation in the semen

Study characteristics			Indication		Sperm retrieval method		Outcomes		
Reference	Design	Subjects and cohort size (N)	Test used for sperm chromatin damage assessment and cut-off values (%)	Paired SDF results in testicular and ejaculated sperm (%)	Sperm retrieval method	Sperm retrieval success and complication rates (%)	Fertilization rate (%)	Clinical pregnancy rate (%)	Ongoing pregnancy or live birth rates[5] (%)
31	Case series	Predominantly normozoospermic infertile men (18) Couples with history of ICSI failure performed with ejaculated sperm	TUNEL (15)	23.6 ± 5.1 (E) and 4.8 ± 3.6 (T) ($p < 0.001$)	TESE and TESA	100 and NR	74.9[1]	44.4[2]	NR
20	Case series	Couples with history of IVF/ICSI failure (68) with ejaculated sperm	TUNEL (20)	NR	TESA	NR	58.0; range: 20–100	40.0	NR
34	Prospective cohort	Oligozoospermic (sperm concentration 5–15 million/ml) infertile men (172) Couples with no history of ICSI failure (Testi-ICSI, $n = 81$ and Ejac-ICSI, $n = 91$)	SCD (30)	40.9 ± 10.2 (E) and 8.3 ± 5.3 (T) ($p < 0.001$)	TESE and TESA	100 and 6.2	69.4 (E) vs. 56.1 (T) ($p = 0.0001$)	40.2 (E) vs. 51.9 (T) (NS)	LBR: 26.4 (E) vs. 46.7 (T) ($p = 0.007$)
35	Case series	Oligozoospermic (sperm concentration <5 million/ml) infertile men (24) Couples with one or more failed IVF or ICSI cycles using ejaculated sperm	TUNEL (7)	24.0 (9% CI: 19–34) (E) and 5.0 (95% CI: 3–7) (T) ($p = 0.001$)	Micro-TESE	100 and NR	54.0	50	50
49	Retrospective cohort	Predominantly oligozoospermic men infertile men*; Testi-ICSI ($n = 148$), Ejac-ICSI ($n = 80$)	SCIT (29)	NR	TESE and TESA	NR	66.0 (E) vs. 57.0 (T) ($p < 0.001$)	27.5 (E) vs. 49.5 (T) ($p < 0.01$)	24.2 (E) vs. 49.8 (T) ($p < 0.05$)

#	Study design	Population	SDF test (threshold, %)	SDF value	Sperm retrieval	Fertilization rate[1] (T and E)	Blastocyst/implantation	Clinical pregnancy	Pregnancy/birth outcome
50	Retrospective cohort	Normozoospermic infertile men (71) Couples with history of ICSI failure using ejaculated sperm (Testi-ICSI, $n = 31$; Ejac-ICSI, $n = 40$)	TUNEL (30)	41.7 ± 8.2 (E)	TESA	100 and NR	74.1 ± 20.7 (T) and 71.1 ± 26.9 (E) (NS)	41.9 (T) and 20.0 (E) ($p = 0.04$)	OPR: 38.7 (T) vs. 15.0 (E) ($p = 0.02$)
51	Prospective cohort; interventions applied in the same patients	Oligozoospermic and normozoospermic infertile men (36) Couples with history of ICSI failure performed with ejaculated sperm	SCD (30)	56.3 ± 15.3 (E)	TESA	100 and NR	46.4 (T) and 47.8 (E) (NS)	38.9 (T) and 13.8 (E) ($p < 0.0001$)	LBR: 38.9 (T) vs. 8.0 (E) ($p < 0.0001$)
52	Prospective cohort[4]	Oligozoospermic and normozoospermic infertile men (102) Couples with no history of ICSI failure (Testi-ICSI, $n = 61$; Ejac-ICSI, $n = 41$)	SCSA (30)	NR	TESA	100 and NR	70.4 (T) vs. 75.0 (E) (NS)	36.0 (T) vs. 14.6 (E) ($p = 0.01$)	LBR: 36.0 (T) vs. 9.8 (E) ($p = 0.001$)
53	Retrospective cohort	Couples with no previous live births and a history of at least two previous failed ICSI cycles with ejaculated sperm (Testi-ICSI, $n = 77$; Ejac-ICSI, $n = 68$)	SCSA (≥25); TUNEL (≥36)	NR	TESE	NR	DFI ≥25 (SCSA): 66.3 (T); 62.9 (E) (NS) DFI ≥36 (TUNEL): 61.2 (T); 57.6 (E) (NS)	DFI ≥25 (SCSA): 18.2 (T); 9.1 (E) ($p < 0.02$) DFI ≥36 (TUNEL): 23.1 (T); 0.0 (E) ($p < 0.02$)	[3]DFI ≥25 (SCSA): 21.7 (T); 9.1 (E) ($p < 0.01$) DFI ≥36 (TUNEL): 20.0 (T); 0 (E) ($p < 0.02$)

*Number of ICSI cycles; E, ejaculated sperm group; Ejac-ICSI, ICSI with ejaculated sperm; LBR, live birth rate; micro-TESE, microdissection testicular sperm extraction; NR, not reported; NS, not significantly different; OPR, ongoing pregnancy rate; SCD, sperm chromatin dispersion test; SCIT, sperm chromatin integrity test, a variation of sperm chromatin structure assay (SCSA); SDF, sperm DNA fragmentation; T, testicular sperm group; Testi-ICSI, ICSI with testicular sperm; TESE, Testicular sperm extraction, TESA, testicular sperm aspiration; TUNEL, terminal deoxyribonucleotide transferase-mediated dUTP nick-end labeling assay

1 2PN fertilization rate with use of testicular sperm; data from previous cycles with use of ejaculated sperm not provided; 2 The authors reported only one pregnancy with ejaculated sperm which miscarried; 3 Cumulative live birth rates reported; 4 Inferred from the study reported data; authors not contacted to provide clarification; 5 Herrero et al. reported the cumulative live birth rate.

pregnancies were achieved, which resulted in 13 deliveries, 5 of which were reported for the ejaculate ICSI group and 8 for the testicular ICSI group. The rates of clinical pregnancy and delivery per embryo transfer according to use of testicular and ejaculate sperm were 47.4 versus 20.8 ($p < 0.05$), and 42.1 versus 20.8 ($p = 0.18$).

Later, in 2011, Hauser et al. studied 13 couples whose male partners had virtual azoospermia or cryptozoospermia [48]. Five couples initially underwent ICSI using testicular sperm, because the males had total azoospermia, and later with ejaculate spermatozoa found after centrifugation. Ejaculate sperm were initially used for ICSI in the remaining eight patients, and in later cycles testicular sperm were used. TESE was performed under general anesthesia, and the retrieved sperm were immediately used for ICSI whereas the remaining specimens cryopreserved for later use. In all, ejaculate sperm ICSI was carried out in 34 cycles, fresh testicular sperm ICSI in nine cycles, and frozen–thawed testicular sperm ICSI in 50 cycles. Both fertilization rate (50.0 percent vs. 38.2 percent, $p < 0.05$) and embryo quality (65.3 percent vs. 53.2 percent, $p < 0.05$) were significantly higher when sperm injection was carried out with fresh or frozen–thawed testicular sperm than with ejaculated sperm ($p < 0.05$). Moreover, implantation rates were higher (p = .04) with fresh testicular sperm (18.1 percent) than with frozen–thawed testicular sperm (5.7 percent) and ejaculated sperm (5.1 percent).

In 2012, Amirjannati et al. assessed ICSI outcomes of 192 men with cryptozoospermia [63]. Ejaculated sperm were used in 208 cycles whereas testicular sperm retrieved by micro-TESE were used in nineteen cycles. The authors showed no differences with regards fertilization rates (60.0 ± 31 percent vs. 68.0 ± 30 percent) and number of good-quality embryos according to use of testicular and ejaculated sperm, respectively, but the authors did not report pregnancy data.

One year later, Ben-Ami et al. studied a cohort of seventeen patients with cryptozoospermia who underwent a total of 116 ICSI cycles [49]. Of these, ICSI with ejaculated sperm was carried out in sixty-eight cycles (58.6 percent) whereas ICSI with testicular sperm was used in forty-eight 48 (41.4 percent) cycles. Testicular sperm extraction was the method for sperm retrieval, performed on the day of oocyte pick-up. Among ICSI cycles with testicular sperm, fresh sperm were used in 31 cycles (64.6 percent), whereas frozen–thawed sperm were used in 17 cycles

(35.4 percent). In this series, higher rates of implantation (20.7 versus 5.7 percent; $p = 0.003$), clinical pregnancy (42.5 versus 15.1 percent; $p = 0.004$), and delivery (27.5 versus 9.4 percent; $p = 0.028$) were achieved with the use of testicular sperm than with ejaculated sperm.

In 2016, Abhyankar et al. aggregated the data of the studies mentioned above and completed a meta-analysis on the rates of fertilization and pregnancy [45]. The authors found that the relative risk (RR) of achieving two pronuclei fertilization (4596 injected oocytes; RR = 0.91; 95 percent CI 0.78–1.06) and pregnancy (272 cycles; RR = 0.53, 95 percent CI 0.19, 1.42) with use of testicular or ejaculated sperm for ICSI was not different, and concluded that testicular sperm should not be recommended in preference over ejaculated sperm in men with severe oligozoospermia or cryptozoospermia. However, a careful examination of the authors' results revealed that they inadvertently inverted the number of pregnancies reported by Bendikson et al. for testicular and ejaculate sperm. This critical mistake inflated the total number of pregnancies in the ejaculate sperm group, thus leading to an erroneous RR calculation. We reassessed the pregnancy results of the meta-analysis by Abhyankar et al. after correcting this incongruency and found a significantly higher pregnancy rate with use of testicular sperm than with ejaculated sperm in men with cryptozoospermia and severe oligozoospermia (272 cycles; RR = 2.51, 95 percent CI 1.54–4.1; $I^2 = 27$ percent; $p = 0.0002$) (Esteves SC, Roque M. Extended indications for sperm retrieval: summary of current literature. F1000Res. 2019 Dec 4;8:F1000 Faculty Rev-2054. doi: 10.12688/f1000research.20564.1.).

Still, in 2016, an additional report investigating the efficacy of use of testicular sperm for ICSI among non-azoospermic men with severe oligozoospermia or cryptozoospermia was published [42]. In a prospective comparative study of 73 patients, Ketabchi used freshly ejaculated sperm for ICSI in 35 couples and sperm retrieved from the epididymis ($n = 18$) or testis ($n = 17$) in the remaining patients [42]. Percutaneous aspiration and micro-TESE were used for epididymal and testicular retrievals, respectively. The author reported that the rates of fertilization (85.7 versus 55.3 percent; $p < 0.001$), good-quality embryo (77.1 versus 39.5 percent; $p < 0.05$), and clinical pregnancy (57.1 versus 31.6 percent, $p < 0.01$) have favored the sperm retrieval group.

In 2017, Cui et al. retrospectively studied a group of 285 patients with cryptozoospermia, in which ejaculated sperm were used in 214 cases whereas testicular sperm were used in 71 cases [43]. Either TESA or TESE were carried out on the day of egg collection to harvest sperm from the seminiferous tubules in patients with no ejaculated sperm available for ICSI after examination of the centrifuged pellet. In this series, there was no difference in fertilization rates between groups (60.6 and 59.6 percent). However, significantly higher rates of good-quality embryo (46.1 versus 36.8 percent; $p = 0.001$), implantation (52.1 versus 30.7 percent; $p < 0.01$), clinical pregnancy (53.6 versus 33.3 percent; $p < 0.01$), and live birth (44.6 versus 27.1 percent; $p = 0.02$) were observed with use of testicular sperm than with ejaculated sperm.

A 2018 systematic review and meta-analysis aggregated the data of the studies included in the meta-analysis of Abhyankar et al. and the reports by Ketabchi and Cui et al. [46]. A total of 578 patients and 761 ICSI cycles were evaluated. In this study, testicular sperm ICSI improved the likelihood of achieving good-quality embryos (RR 1.17, 95 percent CI 1.05–1.30; $p = 0.005$), implantation (RR 1.52, 95 percent CI 1.02–2.26; $p = 0.04$), and pregnancy (RR = 1.74, 95 percent CI 1.20–2.52; $p = 0.004$). These results have been corroborated by Ku et al., who pooled the evidence of the above studies that provided miscarriage and live birth data [64]. The authors included four studies [43,47–49] involving 331 patients and 479 ICSI cycles. In this study, miscarriage rates were not affected by the use of testicular or ejaculated sperm for ICSI (RR = 1.06, 95 percent CI 0.48–2.35), but live birth rates per initiated cycle were increased among couples who had undergone ICSI with testicular sperm (RR = 1.77, 95 percent CI 1.28–2.44; $p = 0.0005$).

Lastly, a 2019 retrospective cohort study assessed ICSI outcomes – according to sperm source and paternal age – in a group of men with cryptozoospermia [44]. In total, 35 patients were included, of whom 18 and 17 had ICSI with ejaculated or testicular sperm, respectively. Testicular sperm was harvested by TESA or micro-TESE, and fresh sperm injections were carried out in the vast majority of patients. In this series, ICSI with testicular sperm increased good-quality embryo rates (63.0 versus 26.2 percent; $p = 0.002$) and clinical pregnancy rates (12.5 versus 71.4 versus12.5 percent; $p = 0.04$) among men older than 35 years. By contrast, ICSI with ejaculated sperm increased fertilization rates (74.7 versus 62.4 percent;

$p = 0.02$) and good-quality embryo rates (50.5 versus 36.6 percent; $p = 0.03$) among patients aged 35 years and younger, albeit clinical pregnancy rates were not affected. In this study, there was no difference in the rates of implantation, miscarriage, and live birth between the groups of testicular and ejaculate sperm ICSI, nor did paternal age affected these outcomes.

In summary, existing evidence from seven retrospective studies and one prospective study, including a total of 613 patients and 799 ICSI cycles, suggest that ICSI with testicular sperm is superior to ICSI with ejaculated sperm to overcome infertility among non-azoospermic men with severe oligozoospermia or cryptozoospermia (Table 8.4). Likewise the case of sperm chromatin damage, Testi-ICSI has been postulated to bypass post-testicular sperm damage during sperm transit through the genital tract. However, randomized, controlled studies are required to determine whether testicular sperm could be recommended as routine practice in non-azoospermic men with low semen quality undergoing ICSI.

8.4.4 Risks to Offspring Health

The increased use of sperm retrieval for ICSI in non-azoospermic men has raised concerns about the health of resulting offspring. On the one hand, ICSI has been associated with possible increased risk of congenital malformations, epigenetic disorders, chromosomal abnormalities, infertility, cancer, delayed psychological and neurological development, and impaired cardiometabolic profile compared with naturally conceived children, probably due to the influence of parental subfertility [3]. On the other hand, data concerning risks and sequelae to offspring health with use of surgically retrieved gametes from azoospermic men are overall reassuring, albeit limited [65–69]. However, no study has yet examined whether ICSI with testicular in preference of ejaculated sperm, when both are available, affects the risk of malformations and long-term health of offspring.

Yet, a few reports indicate that aneuploidy rates might be increased in testicular sperm. An early cohort study published in 2001 included 28 infertile men and assessed sperm abnormalities involving chromosomes 18, X, and Y by FISH (fluorescence *in situ* hybridization) analysis [70]. In this series, the rates of aneuploidy were higher in testicular sperm retrieved from patients with nonobstructive azoospermia (19.6 percent) than that of obstructive

Table 8.4 Characteristics and main outcome measures of studies reporting ICSI outcomes with testicular versus ejaculated sperm in non-azoospermic men with severe oligozoospermia/cryptozoospermia

Study characteristics			Indication		Sperm retrieval method		Outcomes			
Reference	Design		Subjects and cohort size (N)	SDF assessment	Sperm retrieval method	Sperm retrieval success and complication rates (%)	Fertilization rate (%)	Clinical pregnancy rate (%)	Live birth rates (%)	
54	Case series		Severe oligozoospermic (<5 million/ml) infertile men (4) undergoing Testi-ICSI. Couples with a history of multiple failed ICSI cycles with ejaculated sperm; in total, five TESA-ICSI cycles were carried out in the cohort of four patients	No	TESA	100 and NR	67.6	75.0	75.0	
55	Case series		Cryptozoospermic infertile men (16). Couples with history of IVF/ICSI failure (16) with ejaculated sperm; in total, 21 TESA-ICSI cycles were carried out in the cohort of 16 patients	No	Micro-TESE	100 and NR	51.7 (T) vs. 59.9 (E) (NS)	20.8 (E) vs. 47.4 (T) (NS)	20.8 (E) vs. 42.1 (T) (NS)	
56	Prospective cohort		Cryptozoospermic infertile men (13). In total, 93 ICSI cycles (ICSI with ejaculated sperm, n = 34; ICSI with fresh testicular sperm, n = 9; ICSI with frozen–thawed testicular sperm, n = 50) were carried out in the cohort of 13 patients	No	TESE	100 and NR	38.2 (E) vs. 50.0 (T, fresh) vs. 46.7 (T, frozen–thawed)* (p < 0.05, pairwise comparisons between T and E sperm)	14.3 (E) vs. 42.9 (T, fresh) vs. 12.8 (T, frozen–thawed) (NS)	14.3 (E) vs. 42.9 (T, fresh) vs. 12.8 (T, frozen–thawed) (NS)	

58	Case series	Cryptozoospermic infertile men (17) Couples with multiple failed ICSI cycles using ejaculated sperm; in total, 116 ICSI cycles (Testi-ICSI, $n = 48$; Ejac-ICSI, $n = 68$) were carried out in the cohort of 16 patients	No	TESE	100 and NR	38.0 (E) vs. 46.7 (T) (NS)	15.1 (E) vs. 42.5 (T) ($p = 0.004$)	9.4 (E) vs. 27.5 (T) ($p = 0.028$)
60	Prospective cohort	Cryptozoospermic ($<10^3$ sperm/ml) infertile men (73) undergoing ICSI with sperm retrieved from the epididymis or testis (18)	No	PESA and TESE	100 and NR	55.3 (E) vs. 85.7 (T +E) ($p < 0.001$)	31.6 (E) vs. 57.1 (T) ($p < 0.001$)	NR
61	Retrospective cohort	Cryptozoospermic infertile men undergoing Testi-ICSI Couples (285) undergoing ICSI with ejaculated sperm (214) or testicular sperm (71)	No	TESA and TESE	97.9 and NR	59.6 (E) vs. 60.6 (T) (NS)	33.3 (E) vs. 53.6 (T) ($p < 0.01$)	27.1 (E) vs. 44.0 (T) ($p = 0.03$)
64	Retrospective cohort	Cryptozoospermic infertile men (35) undergoing Testi-ICSI; in total, 19 cycles (18 patients) were performed with ejaculated sperm and 19 cycles (17 patients) with testicular sperm	No	TESA and micro-TESE	100 percent and NR	74.7 (E) and 62.4 (T) in men <35 years old ($p = 0.01$); 60.9 (E) and 56.6 (T) in men ≥35 years old (NS)	74.7 (E) and 62.4 (T) in men <35 years old ($p = 0.01$); 60.9 (E) and 56.6 (T) in men ≥35 years old (NS)	44.4 (E) and 52.9 (T) in men <35 years old (NS); 0.0 (E) and 42.9 (T) in men ≥35 years old

E, ejaculated sperm group; Ejac-ICSI, ICSI with ejaculated sperm; LBR, live birth rate; micro-TESE, microdissection testicular sperm extraction; NR, not reported; NS, not significantly different; OPR, ongoing pregnancy rate; SDF, sperm DNA fragmentation; T, testicular sperm group; Testi-ICSI, ICSI with testicular sperm; TESE, Testicular sperm extraction; TESA, testicular sperm aspiration.
*2PN fertilization using motile sperm.

azoospermia patients (8.2 percent), as well as ejaculated sperm from patients with severe oligozoospermia (13.0 percent) (p values not reported). In 2002, Palermo et al. investigated sperm aneuploidy rates in chromosomes 18, 21, X, and Y by FISH in a group of 12 azoospermic patients undergoing ICSI [71]. The authors reported higher aneuploidy rates (11.4 percent) in testicular sperm from patients with nonobstructive azoospermia than epididymal sperm from patients with obstructive azoospermia (1.8 percent; $p = 0.0001$).

In another ICSI cohort study published in 2011, involving 25 patients and 20 controls, Rodrigo et al. compared the incidence of diploidy and disomy in testicular sperm and ejaculated sperm [72]. In this series, controls were men with proven fertility (fertile donors and men undergoing vasectomy), whereas patients were men with either obstructive or nonobstructive azoospermia. Testicular sperm had a higher incidence of aneuploidy (by FISH analysis of chromosomes 13, 18, 21, X, and Y) than ejaculated sperm, in both patients and controls. These results were corroborated by Vozdova et al., who studied a large cohort of sperm by FISH in a group of 17 patients with nonobstructive azoospermia and ten fertile controls [73]. The authors showed that the overall frequencies of disomy and diploidy involving chromosomes 13, 15, 16, 18, 21, 22, X, and Y were 2.86 percent and 0.92 percent in patients and controls, respectively ($p < 0.05$).

In 2012, Moskovtsev et al. reported the first study investigating sperm aneuploidy rates in a cohort of 12 non-azoospermic men with high levels of sperm chromatin damage in the semen [33]. In this series, aneuploidy rates by FISH were increased in testicular sperm compared with ejaculated sperm (12.4 ± 3.7 versus 5.7 ± 1.2 percent; $p < 0.05$), despite the fact that sperm chromatin damage was threefold lower in the former (TUNEL: 13.3 percent ± 7.3 versus 39.7 percent ± 14.8).

By contrast, a 2018 study by Cheung et al. showed no increase in testicular sperm aneuploidy rates [74]. The authors used FISH analysis and whole-exome sequencing molecular karyotype (by next-generation sequencing) to assess sperm aneuploidy in a group of 93 fertile donors and infertile patients. The patient subgroup comprised men with azoospermia (both obstructive and nonobstructive) as well as non-azoospermic subjects with high sperm chromatin damage in the ejaculate. In this series, the overall aneuploidy rate by FISH was 3.6 percent in ejaculated

specimens ($n = 87$), 1.2 percent in epididymal specimens ($n = 2$), and 1.1 percent in testicular specimens ($n = 4$), compared to 0.9 percent in the donor specimens. Next-generation sequencing yielded a total aneuploidy of 11.1 percent in the ejaculated group ($n = 16$), 1.8 percent in the epididymal group ($n = 2$), and 1.5 percent for the testicular group ($n = 4$) ($p < 0.0001$). There was no difference in aneuploidy rates between men with obstructive ($n = 3$) and nonobstructive azoospermia ($n = 3$) (6.7 percent versus 5.1 percent). Furthermore, paired assessments in ejaculated and surgically retrieved testicular specimens of non-azoospermic patients ($n = 3$) with high sperm chromatin damage in semen showed that the rates of aneuploidy (1.3 versus 8.4 percent; $p = 0.02$) were lower in testicular sperm than in ejaculated sperm, respectively.

The results of Cheung et al. are consistent with the observations of Suganuma et al., who used a mouse model to investigate the frequency of aneuploidy and structural chromosome aberrations in testicular and epididymal sperm [75]. The authors used an animal model with a defined chromatin defect owing to a mutation in the Tnp gene. This mutation results in the lack of one of the transitional nuclear proteins (TP), thus making the DNA of cauda epididymal sperm more accessible to intercalating dyes due to increased strand breaks. Transitional proteins replace histones during the final stages of spermiogenesis and are, therefore, critical for chromatin remodeling as they are subsequently replaced by protamines in spermatids [75]. In this study, increased chromosomal structural aberrations such as chromatid breaks, chromatid fragmentations, and chromatid exchanges – rather than aneuploidy – were observed in cauda epididymal sperm from mutant mice, which negatively affected embryo development. By contrast, sperm from the testis and caput epididymis of mutant mice showed similar chromosomal integrity and embryo development potential than the sperm of wild-type mice, thus indicating deterioration of sperm genomic material during epididymal transit, which is related to structural aberrations rather than aneuploidy.

Along these lines, Weng et al. showed that the origin of sperm used for ICSI has no marked influence on embryo aneuploidy rates [76]. The authors investigated 572 embryos using FISH analysis for aneuploidy screening in chromosomes 13, 18, 21, X, and Y. In this series, the frequency of aneuploid embryos was not statistically different when ejaculated sperm (59 percent) was compared with epididymal (52 percent) and testicular sperm (52 percent) from azoospermic men. Furthermore, in a 2019 ICSI study, Figueira et al. performed 24-chromosome genetic testing in 940 trophectoderm biopsies of 362 infertile couples [77]. Sperm injections with ejaculated sperm were carried out in 280 couples, whereas surgically retrieved sperm was used in 82 couples. Of these, 86 cycles were performed in couples whose male partners had high levels of sperm chromatin damage in semen, of which 50 cycles were carried out with ejaculated sperm and 36 cycles with testicular sperm. In this series, the probability of a metaphase II oocyte turning into a euploid blastocyst decreased with female age and use of testicular sperm from men with nonobstructive azoospermia. However, among non-azoospermic men with high sperm chromatin damage, the blastocyst euploid rate per metaphase II oocyte was not differently affected whether ejaculated or testicular sperm were used for ICSI (18.7 percent vs. 18.2 percent, respectively).

The observations mentioned above corroborate the safe utilization of surgically retrieved sperm from non-azoospermic men for ICSI. However, owing to limited data concerning offspring health, continuous monitoring is warranted.

8.5 Conclusions

Sperm retrieval for ICSI in non-azoospermic men seems to be beneficial over ICSI with ejaculated sperm, with overall improvements reported in rates of pregnancy, miscarriage, and live birth. Indications include abnormal levels of sperm chromatin damage

in neat semen, severe oligozoospermia, and crypto-zoospermia. The two most common methods are the percutaneous aspiration and open testicular sperm extraction. The risks of complications are low (<5 percent) but might include serious complications; therefore, interventions should be performed by experienced urologists.

Testicular sperm are preferable to epididymal sperm for ICSI as the rates of nuclear and mitochondrial chromatin abnormalities tend to be lower in testicular specimens. The reasons are not fully understood, but it seems to be related to the increased susceptibility of the sperm DNA from infertile men to damage during the epididymal passage, possibly by endogenous nucleases or ROS. Intracytoplasmic sperm injection using sperm with lower chromatin abnormalities might help to explain the improved reproductive outcome with testicular sperm as consistently reported in various studies. However, other mechanisms involving epigenetic factors might play a role and warrant further investigation.

Notwithstanding the potential benefit of Testi-ICSI for non-azoospermic infertile males and the overall reassuring data concerning the health of the resulting offspring, there are risks involved with sperm retrieval. Thus, identification and treatment of the male factor associated with sperm chromatin damage and severe oligozoospermia/cryptozoospermia might enable natural conception or use of ejaculate sperm for ICSI. The benefits and risks of sperm retrieval for non-azoospermic men should be discussed with the affected patients in light of the existing evidence.

References

1. Palermo GD, Neri QV, Rosenwaks Z. To ICSI or not to ICSI. *Semin Reprod Med* 2015;33:92–102.

2. Palermo G, Joris H, Devroey P, Van Steirteghem AC. Pregnancies after intracytoplasmic injection of single spermatozoon into an oocyte. *Lancet* 1992;340:17–18.

3. Esteves SC, Roque M, Bedoschi G, Haahr T, Humaidan P. Intracytoplasmic sperm injection for male infertility and consequences for offspring. *Nat Rev Urol* 2018;15:535–562.

4. Esteves SC, Miyaoka R, Orosz JE, Agarwal A. An update on sperm retrieval techniques for azoospermic males. *Clinics (Sao Paulo)* 2013;68(Suppl. 1):99–110.

5. Esteves SC. Novel concepts in male factor infertility: clinical and laboratory perspectives. *J Assist Reprod Genet* 2016;33:1319–1335.

6. Esteves SC, Miyaoka R, Agarwal A. Surgical treatment of male infertility in the era of intracytoplasmic sperm injection: new insights. *Clinics (Sao Paulo)* 2011;66:1463–1478.

7. Esteves SC. Clinical management of infertile men with nonobstructive azoospermia. *Asian J Androl* 2015;17: 459–470.

8. Miyaoka R, Esteves SC. Predictive factors for sperm retrieval and sperm injection outcomes in obstructive azoospermia: do etiology, retrieval techniques and gamete source play a role?. *Clinics (Sao Paulo)* 2013;68(Suppl. 1):111–119.

9. Esteves SC, Lee W, Benjamin DJ, et al. Reproductive potential of men with obstructive azoospermia undergoing percutaneous sperm

retrieval and intracytoplasmic sperm injection according to the cause of obstruction. *J Urol* 2013;189:232–237.

10. Nagy ZP, Liu J, Joris H, et al. The result of intracytoplasmic sperm injection is not related to any of the three basic sperm parameters. *Hum Reprod* 1995;10:1123–1129.

11. Strassburger, D, Friedler S, Raziel A, et al. Very low sperm count affects the result of intracytoplasmic sperm injection. *J Assist Reprod Genet* 2000;17:431–436.

12. Mitchell V, Rives N, Albert M, et al. Outcome of ICSI with ejaculated spermatozoa in a series of men with distinct ultrastructural flagellar abnormalities. *Hum Reprod* 2006;21:2065–2074.

13. Verza S Jr, Esteves SC. Sperm defect severity rather than sperm source is associated with lower fertilization rates after intracytoplasmic sperm injection. *Int Braz J Urol* 2008;34:49–56.

14. Krawetz SA. Paternal contribution: new insights and future challenges. *Nat Rev Genet* 2005;6:633–642.

15. Agarwal A, Majzoub A, Esteves SC, et al. Clinical utility of sperm DNA fragmentation testing: practice recommendations based on clinical scenarios. *Transl Androl Urol* 2016;5:935–950.

16. Rima D, Shiv BK, Bhavna Ch, Shilpa B, Saima Kh. Oxidative stress induced damage to paternal genome and impact of meditation and yoga: can it reduce incidence of childhood cancer? *Asian Pac J Cancer Prev* 2016;17:4517–4525.

17. Aitken RJ. DNA damage in human spermatozoa: important contributor to mutagenesis in the offspring. *Transl Androl Urol* 2017;6(4):761–764.

18. McPherson S, Longo FJ. Chromatin structure–function alterations during mammalian spermatogenesis: DNA nicking and repair in elongating spermatids. *Eur J Histochem* 1995;37:109–128.

19. Sotolongo B, Huang TT, Isenberger E, Ward WS. An endogenous nuclease in hamster, mouse, and human spermatozoa cleaves DNA into loop-sized fragments. *J Androl* 2005;26:272–280.

20. Sakkas D, Alvarez JG. Sperm DNA fragmentation: mechanisms of origin, impact on reproductive outcome, and analysis. *Fertil Steril* 2010;93:1027–1036.

21. Muratori M, Tamburrino L, Marchiani S, et al. Investigation on the origin of sperm DNA fragmentation: role of apoptosis, immaturity and oxidative stress. *Mol Med* 2015;21:109–122.

22. Gosálvez J, Lopez-Fernandez C, Fernandez JL, Esteves SC, Johnston SD. Unpacking the mysteries of sperm DNA fragmentation: ten frequently asked questions. *J Reprod Biotechnol Fertil* 2015;4:1–16.

23. Santi D, Spaggiari G, Simoni M. Sperm DNA fragmentation index as a promising predictive tool for male infertility diagnosis and treatment management: meta-analyses. *Reprod Biomed Online* 2018;37(3):315–326.

24. Majzoub A, Arafa M, Mahdi M, et al. Oxidation-reduction potential and sperm DNA fragmentation, and their associations with sperm morphological anomalies amongst fertile and infertile men. *Arab J Urol* 2018;16(1):87–95.

25. Moskovtsev SI, Willis J, White J, Mullen JB. Sperm DNA damage: correlation to severity of semen abnormalities. *Urology* 2009;74:789–793.

26. Belloc S, Benkhalifa M, Cohen-Bacrie M, et al. Sperm deoxyribonucleic acid damage in normozoospermic men is related to age and sperm progressive motility. *Fertil Steril* 2014;101:1588–1593.

27. Esteves SC. Interventions to prevent sperm DNA damage effects on reproduction. *Adv Exp Med Biol* 2019;1166:119–148.

28. Steele EK, McClure N, Maxwell RJ, Lewis SE. A comparison of DNA damage in testicular and proximal epididymal spermatozoa in obstructive azoospermia. *Mol Hum Reprod* 1999;5:831–835.

29. O'Connell M, McClure N, Lewis SE. Mitochondrial DNA deletions and nuclear DNA fragmentation in testicular and epididymal human sperm. *Hum Reprod* 2002;17:1565–1570.

30. Hammoud I, Bailly M, Bergere M, et al. Testicular spermatozoa are of better quality than epididymal spermatozoa in patients with obstructive azoospermia. *Urology* 2017;103:106–111.

31. Greco E, Scarselli F, Iacobelli M, et al. Efficient treatment of infertility due to sperm DNA damage by ICSI with testicular spermatozoa. *Hum Reprod* 2005;20:226–230.

32. Moskovtsev SI, Jarvi K, Mullen JB, et al. Testicular spermatozoa have statistically significantly lower DNA damage compared with ejaculated spermatozoa in patients with unsuccessful oral antioxidant treatment. *Fertil Steril* 2010;93:1142–1146.

33. Moskovtsev SI, Alladin N, Lo KC, et al. A comparison of ejaculated and testicular spermatozoa aneuploidy rates in patients with high sperm DNA damage. *Syst Biol Reprod Med* 2012;58:142–148.

34. Esteves SC, Sanchez-Martin F, Sanchez-Martin P, Schneider DT, Gosalvez J. Comparison of reproductive outcome in oligozoospermic men with high sperm DNA fragmentation undergoing intracytoplasmic sperm injection with ejaculated and testicular sperm. *Fertil Steril* 2015;104:1398–1405.

35. Mehta A, Bolyakov A, Schlegel PN, Paduch DA. Higher pregnancy rates using testicular sperm in men with severe oligospermia. *Fertil Steril* 2015;104:1382–1387.

36. Esteves SC, Roque M, Bradley CK, Garrido N. Reproductive outcomes of testicular versus ejaculated sperm for intracytoplasmic sperm injection among men with high levels of DNA fragmentation in semen: systematic review and meta-analysis. *Fertil Steril* 2017;108:456–467.

37. Bradley CK, McArthur SJ, Gee AJ, et al. Intervention improves assisted conception intracytoplasmic sperm injection outcomes for patients with high levels of sperm DNA fragmentation: a retrospective analysis. *Andrology* 2016;4:903–910.

38. Pabuccu EG, Caglar GS, Tangal S, Haliloglu AH, Pabuccu R. Testicular versus ejaculated spermatozoa in ICSI cycles of normozoospermic men with high sperm DNA fragmentation and previous ART failures. *Andrologia* 2017;49(2).doi: 10.1111/and.12609.

39. Zhang J, Xue H, Qiu F, Zhong J, Su J. Testicular spermatozoon is superior to ejaculated spermatozoon for intracytoplasmic sperm injection to achieve pregnancy in infertile males with high sperm DNA damage. *Andrologia* 2018;51: e13175.

40. Herrero MB, Lusignan MF, Son WY, et al. ICSI outcomes using testicular spermatozoa in non-azoospermic couples with recurrent ICSI failure and no previous live births. *Andrology* 2019;7:281–287.

41. Arafa M, AlMalki A, AlBadr M, et al. ICSI outcome in patients with high DNA fragmentation: testicular versus ejaculated spermatozoa. *Andrologia* 2018;50 (1). doi: 10.1111/and.12835.

42. Ketabchi AA. Intracytoplasmic sperm injection outcomes with freshly ejaculated sperms and testicular or epididymal sperm extraction in patients with idiopathic cryptozoospermia. *Nephrourol Mon* 2016;8:e41375.

43. Cui X, Ding P, Gao G, Zhang Y. Comparison of the clinical outcomes of intracytoplasmic sperm injection between spermatozoa retrieved from testicular biopsy and from ejaculate in cryptozoospermia patients. *Urology* 2017;102:106–110.

44. Yu Y, Wang R, Xi Q, et al. Effect of paternal age on intracytoplasmic sperm injection outcomes in cryptozoospermic men: ejaculated or testicular sperm? *Medicine (Baltimore)* 2019;98(26):e16209.

45. Abhyankar N, Kathrins M, Niederberger C. Use of testicular versus ejaculated sperm for intracytoplasmic sperm injection among men with cryptozoospermia: a meta-analysis. *Fertil Steril* 2016;105:1469–1475.

46. Kang YN, Hsiao YW, Chen CY, Wu CC. Testicular sperm is superior to ejaculated sperm for ICSI in cryptozoospermia: an update systematic review and meta-analysis. *Sci Rep* 2018;8:7874.

47. Bendikson KA, Neri QV, Takeuchi T, et al. The outcome of intracytoplasmic sperm injection using occasional spermatozoa in the ejaculate of men with spermatogenic failure. *J Urol* 2008;180:1060–1064.

48. Hauser R, Bibi G, Yogev L, et al. Virtual azoospermia and cryptozoospermia: fresh/frozen testicular or ejaculate sperm for better IVF outcome?. *J Androl* 2011;32:484–490.

49. Ben-Ami I, Raziel A, Strassburger D, et al. Intracytoplasmic sperm injection outcome of ejaculated versus extracted testicular spermatozoa in cryptozoospermic men. *Fertil Steril* 2013;99:1867–1871.

50. Weissman A, Horowitz E, Ravhon A, et al. Pregnancies and live births following ICSI with testicular spermatozoa after repeated implantation failure using ejaculated spermatozoa. *Reprod Biomed Online* 2008;17:605–609.

51. Miyaoka R, Orosz JE, Achermann AP, Esteves SC. Methods of surgical sperm extraction and implications for assisted reproductive technology success. *Panminerva Med* 2019;61:164–177.

52. Schlegel PN, Li PS. Microdissection TESE: sperm retrieval in non-obstructive azoospermia. *Hum Reprod Update* 1998;4:439.

53. Esteves SC. Microdissection testicular sperm extraction (micro-TESE) as a sperm acquisition method for men with nonobstructive azoospermia seeking fertility: operative and laboratory aspects. *Int Braz J Urol* 2013;39:440.

54. Esteves SC, Varghese AC. Laboratory handling of epididymal and testicular spermatozoa: what can be done to improve sperm injections outcome. *J Hum Reprod Sci* 2012;5:233–243.

55. Esteves SC, Bento FC. Implementation of air quality control in reproductive laboratories in full compliance with the Brazilian Cells and Germinative Tissue Directive. *Reprod Biomed Online* 2013;26:9–21.

56. Esteves SC, Verza Jr S. PESA/TESA/TESE sperm processing. In: Nagy Z, Varghese A, Agarwal A (eds.) *Practical Manual of In Vitro*

Fertilization, 2nd edn. Springer, New York, 2019, pp. 202–220.

57. Nabi A, Khalili MA, Halvaei I, Roodbari F. Prolonged incubation of processed human spermatozoa will increase DNA fragmentation. *Andrologia* 2014;46:374–379.

58. Paoli D, Pelloni M, Lenzi A, Lombardo F. Cryopreservation of sperm: effects on chromatin and strategies to prevent them. *Adv Exp Med Biol* 2019;1166:149–167.

59. Lopes LS, Esteves SC. Testicular sperm for intracytoplasmic sperm injection in non-azoospermic men: a paradigm shift. *Panminerva Med* 2019;61:178–186.

60. Ramasamy R, Yagan N, Schlegel PN. Structural and functional changes to the testis after conventional versus microdissection testicular sperm extraction. *Urology* 2005;65:1190–1194.

61. Komori K, Tsujimura A, Miura H, et al. Serial follow up study of serum testosterone and antisperm antibodies in patients with non-obstructive azoospermia after conventional or microdissection testicular sperm extraction. *Int J Androl* 2004;27:32–36.

62. Esteves SC. Should a couple with failed in vitro fertilization or intracytoplasmic sperm injection and elevated sperm DNA fragmentation use testicular sperm for the next cycle? *Eur Urol Focus* 2018;4:296–298.

63. Amirjannati N, Heidari-Vala H, Akhondi MA, et al. Comparison of intracytoplasmic sperm injection outcomes between spermatozoa retrieved from testicular biopsy and from ejaculation in cryptozoospermic men. *Andrologia* 2012;44(Suppl. 1):704–709.

64. Ku FY, Wu CC, Hsiao YW, Kang YN. Association of sperm source with miscarriage and take-home baby after ICSI in cryptozoospermia: a meta-analysis of testicular and ejaculated sperm. *Andrology* 2018;6:882–889.

65. Bonduelle M, Van Assche E, Joris H, et al. Prenatal testing in ICSI pregnancies: incidence of chromosomal anomalies in 1586 karyotypes and relation to sperm parameters. *Hum Reprod* 2002;17:2600–2614.

66. Belva F, De Schrijver F, Tournaye H, et al. Neonatal outcome of 724 children born after ICSI using non-ejaculated sperm. *Hum Reprod* 2011;26:1752–1758.

67. Tsai CC, Huang FJ, Wang LJ, et al. Clinical outcomes and development of children born after intracytoplasmic sperm injection (ICSI) using extracted testicular sperm or ejaculated extreme severe oligo-astheno-teratozoospermia sperm: a comparative study. *Fertil Steril* 2011;96:561–571.

68. Esteves SC, Agarwal A. Reproductive outcomes, including neonatal data, following sperm injection in men with obstructive and nonobstructive azoospermia: case series and systematic review. *Clinics* 2013;68(1):141–150.

69. Meijerink AM, Ramos L, Janssen AJ, et al. Behavioral, cognitive, and motor performance and physical development of five-year-old children who were born after intracytoplasmic sperm injection with the use of testicular sperm. *Fertil Steril* 2016;106:1673–1682.

70. Levron J, Aviram-Goldring A, Madgar I, et al. Sperm chromosome abnormalities in men with severe male factor infertility who are undergoing in vitro fertilization with intracytoplasmic sperm injection. *Fertil Steril* 2001;76:479–484.

71. Palermo GD, Colombero LT, Hariprashad JJ, Schlegel PN, Rosenwaks Z. Chromosome analysis of epididymal and testicular sperm in azoospermic patients undergoing ICSI. *Hum Reprod* 2002;17:570–575.

72. Rodrigo L, Rubio C, Peinado V, et al. Testicular sperm from patients with obstructive and nonobstructive azoospermia: aneuploidy risk and reproductive prognosis using testicular sperm from fertile donors as control samples. *Fertil Steril* 2011;95:1005–1012.

73. Vozdova M, Heracek J, Sobotka V, Rubes J. Testicular sperm aneuploidy in non-obstructive azoospermic patients. *Hum Reprod* 2012;27:2233–2239.

74. Cheung S, Schlegel PN, Rosenwaks Z, Palermo GD. Revisiting aneuploidy profile of surgically retrieved spermatozoa by whole exome sequencing molecular karyotype. *PLoS ONE* 2019;14:e0210079.

75. Suganuma R, Yanagimachi R, Meistrich ML. Decline in fertility of mouse sperm with abnormal chromatin during epididymal passage as revealed by ICSI. *Hum Reprod* 2005;20: 3101–3108.

76. Weng SP, Surrey MW, Danzer HC, et al. Chromosome abnormalities in embryos derived from microsurgical epididymal sperm aspiration and testicular sperm extraction. *Taiwan J Obstet Gynecol* 2014;53:202–205.

77. Figueira R, Carvalho JF, Bento FC, et al. ICSI using surgically retrieved testicular sperm of non-azoospermic men with high sperm DNA fragmentation index and blastocyst ploidy: a safe approach. Abstracts of the 35th Annual Meeting of the European Society of Human Reproduction and Embryology. *Hum Reprod* 2019;34(1):i1–i543.

Predictors of Positive Surgical Sperm Retrieval in Azoospermic Males

Evaluation of Clinical, Laboratory, and Histopathologic Factors

Kareim Khalafalla, Ahmed H. Almalki, Ahmad Majzoub, and Sandro C. Esteves

9.1 Introduction

The introduction of surgical sperm retrieval in the 1990s has revolutionized the field of male infertility, notably as it provided hope to patients with azoospermia to father their biological children. Since that time, efforts have focused on optimizing the sperm retrieval techniques and searching for predictors of success.

Azoospermia, defined by the absence of sperm in the ejaculate after examination of the centrifuged pellet, occurs in around 1 percent of men of the general population and in up to 12 percent of infertile men [1,2]. Azoospermia can be classified as obstructive or nonobstructive, with nonobstructive azoospermia (NOA) accounting for most cases (60 percent) [1,2]. This can be caused by a wide spectrum of etiologies, some which are severe and untreatable, such as genetic (Klinefelter syndrome and Y chromosome microdeletions), congenital (cryptorchidism), exposure to gonadal toxin (chemotherapy, radiotherapy), post-infection (mumps), trauma, and idiopathic; in some rare occasions NOA can be due to a treatable endocrine disorder such as hypogonadotropic hypogonadism, which is simply testicular failure due to absence of gonadotropin stimulation. Therefore, a detailed history and proper physical exam should be conducted for all azoospermic patients to identify the type and possible etiology for the azoospermia [3].

Several sperm retrieval techniques for NOA patients have been described. Devroey et al. were the first to perform conventional testicular sperm extraction (cTESE) for a group of men with NOA, proving that sperm could be retrieved from patients with testicular failure [3]. Craft and Tsirigotis introduced

a simpler and less invasive modality for sperm retrieval, namely testicular sperm aspiration (TESA) [4]. Nonetheless, the surgical sperm retrieval rate (SRR) with these two modalities did not exceed 50 percent. Aiming to improve the SRR and, at the same time, minimize damage to testicular parenchyma, Schlegel introduced the microsurgical testicular sperm extraction (micro-TESE) technique. This method, which utilizes surgical magnification, allows accurate dissection and sampling of dilated seminiferous tubules, thus avoiding vascular damage or extensive destruction of testicular tissue. While micro-TESE can be considered the gold standard method for sperm retrieval in cases of NOA, its success rates are quite variable, ranging from 35 to 77 percent. This discrepancy in success rates can be a subject of considerable uncertainty to the couple seeking treatment [5–8].

There is no doubt that couples presenting with azoospermia face a considerable burden physically, emotionally, and financially in the process of conceiving a child. Understanding the predictors of successful sperm retrieval would provide crucial information necessary for optimal patient counseling that would allow the couple to choose the best method of treatment for their particular condition.

This chapter aims to review the most important predictors of surgical sperm retrieval for men with NOA. Many factors have been investigated and can be classified for simplicity into clinical, laboratory, and histopathological factors.

9.2 Clinical Evaluation

The etiology of infertility carries important prognostic information, whether it is a genetic cause like

Table 9.1 Predictors of testicular sperm retrieval

Predictor	Effectiveness	Ref.
Klinefelter syndrome	The SRR in patients with Klinefelter syndrome is 30–50 percent Higher pre-retrieval serum testosterone seems to have a favorable effect on the SRR	[10–14]
Cryptorchidism	The SRR for cryptorchid men is believed to be higher than all other men with NOA, with success rates reaching 74 percent.	[13,14]
Varicocele	Varicocele ligation in NOA patients with clinical varicocele has a favorable effect on SRR	[15]
Age	Controversy surrounds the predictive value of patients' age on the sperm retrieval outcome	[16–22]
Testicular volume	Testicular volume has a low or no predictive value for SRR	[23,24]
FSH	FSH has a low-moderate prognostic value for SRR with better results obtained with lower serum FSH values	[25–27]
Inhibin B	Controversy surrounds the predictive value of serum inhibin B levels on the sperm retrieval outcome	[28–31]
Y chromosome microdeletion	The result of Y chromosome microdeletion significantly predicts the sperm retrieval outcome. Patients with AZFc and partial AZFb microdeletions have an SRR of 54.8 percent and 7.1 percent, respectively. AZFa, AZFb, or AZFa/b microdeletions are associated with the worst prognosis and are deemed likely for failure	[32,33]
Surgical technique	The highest SRR is achieved with mTESE, followed by TESE and TESA	[34–36]
Histologic pattern	Hypospermatogenesis carries the best SRR (80–100 percent), followed by maturation arrest (40–80 percent) and Sertoli-cell-only syndrome (4–51 percent)	[37–40]
Medical treatment prior to surgical sperm retrieval	Testicular hyperstimulation with medications such as clomiphene citrate, human chorionic gonadotropin, follicular FSH, or aromatase inhibitors may have a positive effect on the SRR, although with conflicting results.	[41–45]

Klinefelter syndrome or Y chromosome microdeletions, or an acquired one like cryptorchidism, post-cancer treatment, or varicocele [9]. Other clinical factors, such as patient age and testicular size, can also have an impact on the SRR (Table 9.1).

9.2.1 Klinefelter Syndrome

Klinefelter syndrome (KS) is the most commonly encountered genetic abnormality in men with infertility. It is characterized by the presence of a supernumerary X chromosome (47,XXY), which presents in mosaic forms (e.g., 46,XY/47,XXY) that constitutes around 10–15 percent of KS patients or non-mosaic forms (e.g., 47,XXY) that constitutes around 80–90 percent of KS patients [46–48], and to a lesser extent in the form of chromosomal aneuploidies with more

than one extra X chromosomes (e.g., 48,XXXY or 48, XXYY) and structurally abnormal X chromosome due to translocation (e.g., 47,iXqY) [49–52].

Klinefelter syndrome is prevalent in around 3–4 percent of infertile couples and in 10 percent of azoospermic patients [53]. It was once believed that KS patients are sterile, and the only way to father children was through adoption or donor insemination, until further reports starting from the 1980s showed sperm in some cohorts of KS patients, demonstrating the possible presence of spermatogenic foci in their testicles [53,54]. Around 92 percent of non-mosaic KS patients do not produce sperm in their ejaculates [51], while mosaic forms may present with a picture of oligospermia and hence have a less severe form of infertility.

Up to 50 percent of men with KS can have sperm detected during sperm retrieval using TESE/micro-

TESE [10]. Others have reported a lower SRR; Garolla et al. evaluated 111 non-mosaic azoospermic KS patients retrospectively and reported a 34 percent SRR [11]. Despite that, the SSR in KS patients is believed by some authors to be equivalent to or slightly less than the SRR for men with NOA secondary to other causes [12].

Predictive factors for sperm retrieval in KS patients have been a debatable issue for some time, with no real consensus available to draw solid conclusions. Many factors have been investigated, such as age, testes volume, serum levels of testosterone, luteinizing hormone (LH), and presence of mosaicism, without any clear recommendation [55–57].

Patients younger than 30–35 years old are believed to have a better chance for sperm retrieval compared to older men [55–57]. This has been explained by the progressive testicular degeneration that occurs as KS patients age. On the contrary, other authors did not find any difference in retrieval rate between young and older patients with KS [58,59].

Another factor is the serum testosterone level before surgical sperm retrieval. Sabbaghian et al. observed that higher testosterone levels were associated with better SRR using micro-TESE in KS patients. The authors explained that KS patients presenting with testicular failure usually have hyperplastic Leydig cells, which are unable to produce enough testosterone. Since intratesticular testosterone is vital for normal spermatogenesis, the authors suggested that a serum level testosterone above 2.95 ng/ml may indicate the presence of focal areas of sperm production [60].

Ramasamy et al. reported improved SRR in KS patients who received gonadotropin therapy, suggesting that exogenous gonadotropins decrease the endogenous levels, thus causing a reset-like mechanism for the hormonal receptors in the testicular Sertoli and Leydig cells, leading to later improved function [61]. Another retrospective study by Ramasamy et al. investigating the effects of medical therapy on the sperm retrieval outcomes in KS patients found that men with low baseline testosterone levels receiving treatment before sperm retrieval had a significantly higher SRR when their testosterone levels post-medical therapy were improved above 250 ng/dl compared to men who did not. The authors suggested that a better response to medical therapy may predict the sperm retrieval outcome in KS patients [62].

9.2.2 Cryptorchidism

Cryptorchidism is a common childhood malformation occurring in 3 percent of full-term infants and to a greater extent in preterm infants. It is associated with infertility, hernia, testicular torsion, and tumors. Controversy is still present on whether the age of correction and testes volume is considered as a combined predictor for sperm retrieval [63]. In general, the SRR for cryptorchid men is believed to be higher than for all other men with NOA, with success rates reaching 74 percent [13,14].

Raman and Schlegel investigated 38 cryptorchid patients out of 275 NOA patients and observed significantly higher SRR in patients who had their orchiopexy performed before the age of 10 years compared to a later age of correction [14]. Wiser et al. found no significance with regards to the age of orchiopexy in a group of 40 patients [64]. This latter finding was also echoed by Glina et al. [65].

9.2.3 Varicocele

Varicocele is the most common correctable cause of male infertility, prevalent in about 25–35 percent of infertile men and 5 percent of men with NOA [66,67].

The outcome of varicocelectomy on azoospermic patients was investigated by Mattews et al., who observed that sperm could become detectable in the ejaculate of azoospermic patients following varicocelectomy, thereby avoiding testicular sperm retrieval at the time of intracytoplasmic sperm injection (ICSI). Even in patients who remain azoospermic, varicocelectomy was found to improve the SRR at the time of ICSI [68].

Inci et al. evaluated 96 patients with varicocele and NOA. These authors compared the surgical sperm retrieval outcomes in two groups of patients: 66 patients who underwent varicocelectomy 5–6 months prior to ICSI; and 30 patients who went directly to ICSI. The results showed a statistically significant improvement in the SRR in the group who underwent varicocelectomy compared to the untreated group. It is worth mentioning, however, that there were no significant differences in embryo quality, abortion rate, or live birth rate between the groups [69].

Others did not show a significant improvement in the success rates of sperm retrieval by micro-TESE following varicocelectomy in NOA patients with varicocele. Schlegel et al. examined 31 NOA patients who underwent varicocelectomy and showed that sperm appeared in the ejaculate of 22 percent of patients in at least one semen analysis following surgery, while only 9.6 percent of them produced viable sperm at the time of ICSI [70]. In this study, however, the authors included men with clinical as well as subclinical varicocele.

A systematic review and meta-analysis by Esteves et al. examined 18 studies, including 468 patients with NOA and clinical varicocele. The authors reported a 2.6-fold increase in SRR in treated versus untreated groups, with 44 percent of patients having enough viable sperm in their ejaculate to avoid testicular sperm retrieval [15].

9.2.4 Age

Advancing age is believed to be a negative predictor for pregnancy rates in general, and surgical sperm recovery rates specifically. Younger patients undergoing surgical sperm retrieval tend to have better results with ICSI than do older patients [16–18]. The explanation for this is that as men age, the testicular areas of spermatogenesis decrease, in concordance with a reduction in testes size and seminiferous tubule length [19,20]. Despite this, some studies failed to confirm these observations, thus making age a debatable predictive factor for sperm retrieval.

Ramasamy et al. did not observe any adverse effects for age on sperm retrieval. The authors highlighted that most older patients had acquired causes of NOA, whereas the causes were predominately congenital in the younger age group [21]. Similarly, Enatsu et al., in a study of 329 men with NOA undergoing surgical sperm retrieval and ICSI, did not find a significant adverse effect of patient age on SRR [22].

9.2.5 Testicular Volume

It is generally believed that testicular size reflects the state of spermatogenesis, suggesting that smaller testes may predict worse histopathology and hence lower SRR, while larger testes may have a better SRR [71–73].

As such, some authors tried to identify cut-off values for the testicular size that would predict surgical sperm retrieval. Macaroni et al. reported a 30 percent SRR with micro-TESE when the testes size was less than 8 ml [74] , whereas Bromage et al. reported a 29 percent SRR with TESE when the testes size was less than 4 ml [75]. Ziaee et al. reported that a positive

SRR can be expected in patients with an average testes size of 17.5 ml, while a negative SRR will be obtained with an average testes size of 5.7 ml, with a positive predictive value of 80 percent and a negative predictive value of 96.9 percent with regards to testicular volume and successful SRR (area under the curve [AUC] = 0.95) [76]. However, the authors used different surgical sperm retrieval methods, thereby suggesting improbability of their results. On the other hand, considerable evidence has failed to confirm a significant effect of testicular size on SRR.

A meta-analysis by Hao et al. including five studies with a total of 1764 patients with NOA undergoing surgical sperm retrieval reported that testicular volume had a low predictive value for SRR. The pooled odds ratio was 1.98 (95 percent CI: 1.11–3.53), with sensitivity of 0.8 (95 percent CI: 0.78–0.83), specificity of 0.35 (95 percent CI: 0.32–0.39), positive likelihood ratio of 1.49 (95 percent CI: 0.94–2.36), and negative likelihood ratio of 0.73 (95 percent CI: 0.60–0.88) (AUC = 0.638) [23].

Bryson et al. conducted a retrospective review of 1127 NOA patients who underwent micro-TESE followed by ICSI. The authors divided patients into three groups according to testes size: group 1: testis size <2 ml; group 2: testis size 2–10 ml; group 3, testis size ≥10 ml. The SRR rate was similar among the three groups: group 1, 54.7 percent; group 2, 56.2 percent; and group 3, 55.1 percent. Moreover, no significant differences were observed with regards to pregnancy rates or live births between patients from the three groups who had a positive sperm retrieval outcome [24].

9.3 Laboratory Predictors

Laboratory predictors of SRR have been based on tests that evaluate the function of the hypothalamic–pituitary–gonadal axis, such as FSH, testosterone, anti-Müllerian hormone (AMH), inhibin, and the genetic detection of chromosomal abnormalities such as KS, chromosomal translocations, and Y chromosome microdeletions.

9.3.1 Follicle-Stimulating Hormone

Spermatogenesis is a complex process that is intricately orchestrated by the proper functioning of the hypothalamic–pituitary–gonadal system. Follicle-stimulating hormone is a pituitary glycoprotein produced in response to gonadotropin-releasing hormone stimulation from the hypothalamus. It produces its action by binding to the testicular Sertoli cells, stimulating them to secrete inhibin B, activin, and other nutrients essential for spermatogenesis. Follicle-stimulating hormone is one of the important hormones that is considered as a predictor for testicular function and, therefore, a predictor for sperm retrieval. While it is believed that, in general, FSH concentration is inversely related to SRR, no agreed-upon cut-off value can guarantee the finding of sperm during sperm retrieval [41,77,78].

Ramasamy et al. evaluated the sperm retrieval outcomes of 792 patients undergoing micro-TESE. The pre-procedure FSH levels were divided into four groups: group 1, <15 IU/ml; group 2, 15–30 IU/ml; group 3, 31–45 IU/ml; and group 4, >45 IU/ml. The authors reported a statistically significantly higher SRR in groups 2 (60 percent), 3 (67 percent), and 4 (60 percent) in comparison to group 1 (51 percent) [25]. By contrast, Chen et al. identified an FSH value of 19.4 IU/ml above which no sperm recovery could be expected on retrieval procedures [26].

A systematic review and meta-analysis by Yang et al., including 11 studies and 1350 patients, was conducted to examine the predictive value of FSH on a positive SRR. The authors found FSH to have a moderate diagnostic value as an independent predictor for SRR in patients with NOA (pooled diagnostic odds ratio 3.99 [95 percent CI: 2.33–6.83] and an AUC of 0.72 ± 0.04) . The authors, however, observed significant heterogeneity that was mainly influenced by the region of the included studies and the age of the patients. The diagnostic odds ratio was four times higher in studies from East Asia compared with other regions, and also four times higher in patients younger than 33 years in comparison to older patients [27].

9.3.2 Inhibin B

Inhibin B, along with other glycoproteins such as activins and anti-Müllerian hormone, is considered negative feedback regulators of the hypothalamic–pituitary–gonadal axis. Inhibin B levels decrease in cases of testes dysfunction and hypospermatogenesis. These hormones have been measured in both blood plasma and semen, and assessed as predictors of sperm recovery in patients with NOA [79].

Some reports strongly advocate its role as a predictor of sperm retrieval with a sensitivity and specificity reaching above 80 percent [28,29]. However, most published data do not consider inhibin B as a predictive factor at all. One study by Tunc et al. investigating 52 NOA patients showed no significant differences in SRR based on serum inhibin levels [30]. Another study, by Vernaeve et al., showed the same findings from 185 patients with NOA undergoing sperm retrieval. The authors measured serum inhibin B before the procedure and divided the patients into groups according to whether sperm was recovered or not. The mean serum inhibin was 37.3 ± 5.4 pg/ml in the group of patients in whom sperm was recovered, and 44.9 ± 7.7 pg/ml in the counterpart with failed retrieval. The authors concluded that inhibin B, alone or combined with FSH, is of limited predictive value in sperm recovery in NOA patients [31].

Mitchell et al., in a study comparing the SRR in 139 azoospermic patients, found that seminal levels of inhibin or AMH did not influence the retrieval outcome [80].

9.3.3 Y Chromosome Microdeletion

Y chromosome microdeletions were first described by Tiepolo and Zuffradi, and are recognized as significant causes of spermatogenic dysfunction and male infertility. These deletions are localized to a group of genes located in the heterochromatic and adjacent euchromatic regions of the Y chromosome, which is also known as the Azoospermia Factor (AZF). Three non-overlapping regions of the Y chromosome, termed AZFa, AZFb, and AZFc, significantly contribute to spermatogenesis; microdeletions within these regions would lead to primary testicular insufficiency characterized by azoospermia or severe oligozoospermia.

AZFa microdeletions carry the worst fertility prognosis as they are associated with Sertoli-cell-only syndrome (SCOS), while AZFb deletions are usually associated with maturation arrest [81,82]. Testing for Y chromosome microdeletions is crucial in azoospermic patients before sperm retrieval as the test result carries prognostic information. AZFa, AZFb, or AZFa/b microdeletions are associated with the worst prognosis and are deemed likely for failure. Patients with AZFc and partial AZFb (associated or not with AZFc) microdeletions have a surgical SRR of 54.8 percent and 7.1 percent, respectively. Moreover, AZFc patients are not necessarily azoospermic and may be candidates for ICSI using sperm from their ejaculate [32,33].

9.3.4 Surgical Technique

Various methods for surgical sperm retrieval have been identified; namely percutaneous TESA, cTESE, and micro-TESE. Each method has its pros and cons, and are described in detail in Chapter 6 [83].

Micro-TESE is considered superior to other methods as it allows a magnified visualization of the seminiferous tubules, allowing selective identification and selection of dilated opaque tubules suspected of containing sperm [34,35].

Many systematic reviews and meta-analyses have been published discussing and comparing the different SRR between methods of surgical sperm retrieval. Deruyver et al., in a systematic review that included seven studies comparing cTESE and micro-TESE, reported an overall SRR ranging between 16.7 and 45 percent in the conventional arm compared to 42.9–63 percent in the microdissection arm. One point noted in this review is that SRR with micro-TESE was significantly higher in Sertoli-cell-only cases of NOA, suggesting that focal areas of spermatogenesis identified microscopically aided in these results. In cases of maturation arrest or hypospermatogensis, the micro-TESE outcome was less advantageous [84].

Another meta-analysis and systematic review by Bernie et al. included 15 studies comparing the three methods of retrieval: TESA, cTESE, and micro-TESE. Data from 1890 patients was analyzed, showing superiority for micro-TESE regarding the SRR (52 percent) in direct comparison to cTESE (35 percent), equating to 1.5 times higher likelihood of sperm retrieval with micro-TESE than cTESE. On the other hand, sperm were twice as likely to be retrieved with cTESE (56 percent) when compared to TESA (28 percent) [36].

9.3.5 Histological Pattern

Testicular histology is believed to be the single most significant predictive factor for successful sperm recovery. Nonetheless, in order to obtain such information, a diagnostic testicular biopsy is required. This practice has not been endorsed by international societies as the biopsy may have a negative influence on testicular function and hence might alter the outcome of the subsequent sperm retrieval. Furthermore, the diagnostic biopsy does not provide an overall view of the histopathologic pattern, which is often variable in the majority of cases. It is believed that hypospermatogenesis carries the best SRR (80–100 percent), followed by maturation arrest (40–80 percent); SCOS has the worst SRR, as low as 4 percent in some studies and as high as 51 percent in others [37–40].

9.3.6 Medical Treatment Prior to Sperm Retrieval

Existing evidence suggests that the sperm retrieval outcome may be improved with hormonal stimulation prior to surgery. While this notion may seem not to be reasonable, especially in men with testicular failure as they will already present with elevated gonadotropins, the concept of hyperstimulating the testes remains an appealing maneuver. Studies show that increasing serum testosterone and FSH levels with estrogen receptor modulators can be associated with a better SRR in patients with NOA [42,43]. Shiraishi investigated the utility of human chorionic gonadotropin injections in patients with previously negative sperm retrieval and reported a positive outcome with micro-TESE in 20 percent of patients six months after the initial procedure [44]. Some authors advised the administration of exogenous FSH as a treatment modality to increase surgical SRRs. Aydos et al. investigated 108 NOA patients with normal FSH levels subjected to testicular sperm retrieval. Recombinant FSH three times a week for three months was given to 63 patients while the remaining 45 patients served as controls. The authors observed a significant improvement in SRR in treated patients (64 percent) compared to untreated patients (33 percent) ($p < 0.01$) [41].

Contrary to this, one large retrospective study of 1054 NOA patients undergoing micro-TESE failed to find any improvement in SRR in patients who received preoperative treatment with aromatase inhibitors, clomiphene citrate, or human chorionic gonadotropin compared to those who did not receive any treatment [45].

9.4 Future Directives in the Predictors of Testicular Sperm Retrieval

Advancements in diagnostic technologies have allowed for the search for new biomarkers that can be used to better understand the etiology of azoospermia and at the same time help in predicting the likelihood of successful sperm retrieval. Examples of these biomarkers include CD133 and CD24, ADAMTS1 and ADAMTS5, and PIWI-interacting RNA (piRNA). CD133 and CD24 are stem cell biomarkers that were found to be significantly lower in NOA patients compared with an OA group. Furthermore, the gene expression of CD133 and CD24 was found to be significantly different among the various histopathologies of NOA patients, being worse in patients with SCO, suggesting that they can be used as potential biomarkers for sperm retrieval [85]. ADAMTS1 and ADAMTS5 are metalloproteinases known to be responsible for the degradation of extracellular matrix (ECM) proteins. Aydos et al. investigated ADAMTS1 and ADAMTS5 in Sertoli cell cultures and ejaculates of patients with NOA, obstructive azoospermia, and a fertile control group. The authors observed that the expression of ADAMTS1 and ADAMTS5 in Sertoli cell cultures was significantly lower in patients with NOA ($2.56\times$ and $2.10\times$ lower, respectively) compared with the obstructive azoospermia group. The picture was similar when comparing the expression of ADAMTS1 and ADAMTS5 in ejaculates of NOA patients with those of the control group [86]. piRNA is a subgroup of small RNAs expressed in germ cells, and plays an important role in regulating spermatogenesis. Cao et al. explored 18 324 piRNAs obtained from testicular tissue samples of 10 NOA patient undergoing micro-TESE. The authors reported discrepancies in the expression of piRNAs between patients with successful and unsuccessful sperm retrieval. However, they particularly identified 553 piRNAs that were absent in patients with unsuccessful SSR and which were abundantly expressed in patients with successful SSR, suggesting that they might be used as potential markers for successful SSR [87].

9.5 Conclusion

Much controversy still surrounds the factors that could predict successful sperm retrieval in patients with NOA. The heterogeneity of the methodologies used in the conducted studies could be considered as one good example of this controversy. It is important to remember the variable presentation that men with NOA tend to have, and the fact that in many instances the etiology remains unknown.

Out of all the factors that have been investigated, testicular histology and, to a lesser extent, serum FSH levels, seem to be most influential in predicting the likelihood of successful sperm retrieval. Advancements in the diagnostic modalities of this field of medicine are warranted to improve our understanding of the complex pathophysiologic mechanisms leading to azoospermia and to perhaps help us find more accurate predictors of sperm retrieval.

References

1. Willott GM. Frequency of azoospermia. *Forensic Sci Int* 1982;20:9–10.

2. Jarow JP, Espeland MA, Lipshultz LI. Evaluation of the azoospermic patient. *J Urol* 1989;142:62–65.

3. Esteves SC. Clinical management of infertile men with nonobstructive azoospermia. *Asian J Androl* 2015;17 (3):459–470.

4. Craft I, Tsirigotis M, Courtauld E, Farrer-Brown G. Testicular needle aspiration as an alternative to biopsy for the assessment of spermatogenesis. *Hum Reprod* 1997;12:1483–1487.

5. Ishikawa T, Nose R, Yamaguchi K, et al. Learning curves of microdissection testicular sperm extraction for nonobstructive azoospermia. *Fertil Steril* 2010;94:1008–1011.

6. Okada H, Dobashi M, Yamazaki T, et al. Conventional versus microdissection testicular sperm extraction for nonobstructive azoospermia. *J Urol* 2002;168:1063–1067.

7. Ramasamy R, Yagan N, Schlegel PN. Structural and functional changes to the testis after conventional versus microdissection testicular sperm extraction. *Urology* 2005;65:1190–1194.

8. Tsujimura A, Matsumiya K, Miyagawa Y, et al. Prediction of successful outcome of microdissection testicular sperm extraction in men with idiopathic nonobstructive azoospermia. *J Urol* 2004;172:1944–1947.

9. Esteves SC, Miyaoka R, Agarwal A. An update on the clinical assessment of the infertile male. *Clinics (Sao Paulo)* 2011;66:691–700. Erratum in: *Clinics (Sao Paulo)* 2012;67:203.

10. Corona G, Pizzocaro A, Lanfranco F, et al. Sperm recovery and ICSI outcomes in Klinefelter syndrome: a systematic review and meta-analysis. *Hum Reprod Update* 2017;23:265–275.

11. Garolla A, Selice R, Menegazzo M, et al. Novel insights on testicular volume and testosterone replacement therapy in Klinefelter patients undergoing testicular sperm extraction: a retrospective

clinical study. *Clin Endocrinol (Oxf)* 2018;88:711–718.

12. Schlegel PN. Nonobstructive azoospermia: a revolutionary surgical approach and results. *Semin Reprod Med* 2009;27:165–170.

13. Ramasamy R, Padilla WO, Osterberg EC, et al. A comparison of models for predicting sperm retrieval before microdissection testicular sperm extraction in men with nonobstructive azoospermia. *J Urol* 2013;189(2):638–642

14. Raman JD, Schlegel PN. Testicular sperm extraction with intracytoplasmic sperm injection is successful for the treatment of nonobstructive azoospermia associated with cryptorchidism. *J Urol* 2003;170(4 Pt 1):1287–1290.

15. Esteves SC, Miyaoka R, Roque M, Agrawal A. Outcome of varicocele repair in men with nonobstructive azoospermia: systemic review and meta-analysis. *Asian J Androl* 2016;18:246–253.

16. Klonoff-Cohen HS, Natarajan L. The effect of advancing paternal age on pregnancy and live birth rates in couples undergoing in vitro fertilization or gamete intrafallopian transfer. *Am J Obstet Gynecol* 2004;191:507–514.

17. Aitken RJ, Baker MA Oxidative stress, sperm survival and fertility control. *Mol Cell Endocrinol* 2006;250:66–69.

18. Evenson DP, Wixon R Clinical aspects of sperm DNA fragmentation detection and male infertility. *Theriogenology* 2006;65:979–991.

19. Belloc S, Cohen-Bacrie P, Benkhalifa M, et al. Effect of maternal and paternal age on pregnancy and miscarriage rates after intrauterine insemination. *Reprod Biomed Online* 2008;17 (3):392–397.

20. Frattarelli JL, Miller KA, Miller BT, Elkind-Hirsch K, Scott RT Jr. Male age negatively impacts embryo development and reproductive outcome in donor oocyte assisted reproductive technology cycles. *Fertil Steril* 2008;90(1):97–103.

21. Ramasamy R, Trivedi NN, Reifsnyder JE, et al. Age does not adversely affect sperm retrieval in men undergoing microdissection testicular sperm extraction. *Fertil Steril* 2014;101:653–655.

22. Enatsu N, Miyake H, Chiba K, Fujisawa M. Predictive factors of successful sperm retrieval on microdissection testicular sperm extraction in Japanese men. *Reprod Med Biol* 2016;15:29–33.

23. Li H, Chen LP, Yang J, et al. Predictive value of FSH, testicular volume, and histopathological findings for the sperm retrieval rate of microdissection TESE in nonobstructive azoospermia: a meta-analysis. *Asian J Androl* 2018;20(1):30–36.

24. Bryson CF, Ramasamy R, Sheehan M, et al. Severe testicular atrophy does not affect the success of microdissection testicular sperm extraction. *J Urol* 2014;191 (1):175–178.

25. Ramasamy R, Lin K, Gosden LV, et al. High serum FSH levels in men with nonobstructive azoospermia does not affect success of microdissection testicular sperm extraction. *Fertil Steril* 2009;92(2):590–593.

26. Chen SC, Hsieh JT, Yu HJ, Chang HC. Appropriate cut-off value for follicle-stimulating hormone in azoospermia to predict spermatogenesis. *Reprod Biol Endocrinol* 2010;8:108.

27. Yang Q, Huang YP, Wang HX, et al. Follicle-stimulating hormone as a predictor for sperm retrieval rate in patients with nonobstructive azoospermia: a systematic review and meta-analysis. *Asian J Androl* 2015;17 (2):281–284.

28. Bohring C, Schroeder-Printzen I, Weidner W, Krause W. Serum levels of inhibin B and follicle-stimulating hormone may predict successful sperm retrieval in men with azoospermia who are undergoing testicular sperm extraction. *Fertil Steril* 2002; 78(6):1195–1198.

29. Ballesca JL, Balasch J, Calafell JM, et al. Serum inhibin B determination is predictive of successful testicular sperm extraction in men with non-obstructive azoospermia. *Hum Reprod* 2000;15(8):1734–1738.

30. Tunc L, Kirac M, Gurocak S, et al. Can serum Inhibin B and FSH levels, testicular histology and volume predict the outcome of testicular sperm extraction in patients with non-obstructive azoospermia? *Int Urol Nephrol* 2006;38(3–4):629–635.

31. Vernaeve V, Tournaye H, Schiettecatte J, et al. Serum inhibin B cannot predict testicular sperm retrieval in patients with non-obstructive azoospermia. *Hum Reprod* 2002;17:971–976.

32. Shefi S, Turek PJ. Sex chromosome abnormalities and male infertility: a clinical perspective. In: De Jonge C, Barrat C (eds.) *The Sperm Cell Production, Maturation, Fertilization, Regeneration.* Cambridge University Press, Cambridge, 2006, pp. 261–278.

33. Stahl PJ, Masson P, Mielnik A, et al. A decade of experience emphasizes that testing for Y microdeletions is essential in American men with azoospermia and severe oligozoospermia. *Fertil Steril* 2010;94(5):1753–1756.

34. Ramasamy R, Yagan N, Schlegel PN. Structural and functional changes to the testis after conventional versus microdissection testicular sperm extraction. *Urology* 2005;65 (6):1190–1194.

35. Esteves SC. Microdissection testicular sperm extraction (micro-TESE) as a sperm

acquisition method for men with nonobstructive azoospermia seeking fertility: operative and laboratory aspects. *Int Braz J Urol* 2013;39(3):440.

36. Bernie AM, Mata DA, Ramasamy R, Schlegel PN. Comparison of microdissection testicular sperm extraction, conventional testicular sperm extraction, and testicular sperm aspiration for nonobstructive azoospermia: a systematic review and meta-analysis. *Fertil Steril* 2015; 104(5):1099–1103.

37. Meng MV, Cha IM, Ljung BM, Turek PJ. Relationship between classic histological pattern and sperm findings on fine needle aspiration map in infertile men. *Hum Reprod* 2000;15 (9):1973–1977.

38. Glina S, Soares JB, Antunes N, Jr., et al. Testicular histopathological diagnosis as a predictive factor for retrieving spermatozoa for ICSI in non-obstructive azoospermic patients. *Int Braz J Urol* 2005; 31(4):338–341.

39. Ramasamy R, Schlegel PN. Microdissection testicular sperm extraction: effect of prior biopsy on success of sperm retrieval. *J Urology* 2007;177(4):1447–1449.

40. Esteves SC, Agarwal A. Re: Sperm retrieval rates and intracytoplasmic sperm injection outcomes for men with non-obstructive azoospermia and the health of resulting offspring. *Asian J Androl* 2014;16(4):642.

41. Aydos K, Unlu C, Demirel LC, Evirgen O, Tolunay O. The effect of pure FSH administration in non-obstructive azoospermic men on testicular sperm retrieval. *Eur J Obstet Gynecol Reprod Biol* 2003;108(1):54–58.

42. Moein MR, Tabibnejad N, Ghasemzadeh J. Beneficial effect of tamoxifen on sperm recovery in infertile men with nonobstructive azoospermia. *Andrologia* 2012; 44(1):194–198.

43. Hussein A, Ozgok Y, Ross L, Rao P, Niederberger C. Optimization of spermatogenesis-regulating hormones in patients with non-obstructive azoospermia and its impact on sperm retrieval: a multicentre study. *BJU Int* 2013;111:E110–E114.

44. Shiraishi K, Ohmi C, Shimabukuro T, Matsuyama H. Human chorionic gonadotropin treatment prior to microdissection testicular sperm extraction in non-obstructive azoospermia. *Hum Reprod* 2012;27:331–339.

45. Reifsnyder JE, Ramasamy R, Husseini J, Schlegel PN. Role of optimizing testosterone before microdissection testicular sperm extraction in men with nonobstructive azoospermia. *J Urol* 2012;188:532–536.

46. Bojesen A, Juul S, Gravholt CH. Prenatal and postnatal prevalence of Klinefelter syndrome: a national registry study. *J Clin Endocrinol Metab* 2003;88 (2):622–626.

47. Friedler S, Raziel A, Strassburger D, et al. Outcome of ICSI using fresh and cryopreserved–thawed testicular spermatozoa in patients with non-mosaic Klinefelter's syndrome. *Hum Reprod* 2001;16 (12):2616–2620.

48. Lanfranco F, Kamischke A, Zitzmann M, Nieschlag E. Klinefelter's syndrome. *Lancet* 2004;364:273–283.

49. Bonomi M, Rochira V, Pasquali D, et al. Klinefelter syndrome (KS): genetics, clinical phenotype and hypogonadism. *J Endocrinol Invest* 2017;40:123–134.

50. Forti G, Corona G, Vignozzi L, Krausz C, Maggi M Klinefelter's syndrome: a clinical and therapeutic update. *Sexual Dev* 2010;4:249–258.

51. Franik S, Hoeijmakers Y, D'Hauwers K, et al. Klinefelter syndrome and fertility: sperm preservation should not be offered to children with Klinefelter syndrome. *Hum Reprod* 2016;31:1952–1959.

52. Hamada AJ, Esteves SC, Agarwal A. A comprehensive review of genetics and genetic testing in azoospermia. *Clinics (Sao Paulo)* 2013;68(1):39–60.

53. Foresta C, Galeazzi C, Bettalla A, et al. Analysis of meiosis in intratesticular germ cells from subjects affected by classic Klinefelter's syndrome. *J Clin Endocrinol Metab* 1999;84:3807–3810.

54. Sciurano RB, Luna Hisano CV, Rahn MI, et al. Focal spermatogenesis originates in euploid germ cells in classical Klinefelter patients. *Hum Reprod* 2009;24:2353–2361.

55. Ferhi K, Avakian R, Griveau JF, Guille F. Age as only predictive factor for successful sperm recovery in patients with Klinefelter's syndrome. *Andrologia* 2009;41:84–87.

56. Ramasamy R, Ricci JA, Palermo GD, et al. Successful fertility treatment for Klinefelter's syndrome. *J Urol* 2009;182:1108–1113.

57. Bakircioglu ME, Ulug U, Erden HF. Klinefelter syndrome: does it confer a bad prognosis in treatment of nonobstructive azoospermia?. *Fertil Steril* 2011;95:1696–1699.

58. Plotton I, Giscard d'Estaing S, Cuzin B, et al. Preliminary results of a prospective study of testicular sperm extraction in young versus adult patients with nonmosaic 47, XXY Klinefelter syndrome. *J Clin Endocrinol Metab* 2015;100:961–967.

59. Mehta A, Bolyakov A, Roosma J, Schlegel PN, Paduch DA. Successful testicular sperm retrieval in adolescents with Klinefelter syndrome treated with at least 1 year of topical testosterone and aromatase

inhibitor. *Fertil Steril* 2013;100:970–974.

60. Sabbaghian M, Modarresi T, Hosseinifar et al. Comparison of sperm retrieval and intracytoplasmic sperm injection outcome in patients with and without Klinefelter syndrome. *Urology* 2014;83:107–110.

61. Ramasamy R, Lin K, Gosden LV, et al. High serum FSH levels in men with nonobstructive azoospermia does not affect success of microdissection testicular sperm extraction. *Fertil Steril* 2009;92:590–593.

62. Ramasamy R, Ricci JA, Palermo GD, et al. Successful fertility treatment for Klinefelter's syndrome. *J Urol* 2009;182:1108–1113.

63. Garrone G, Liguori R. Distopias testiculares e malformacoes genitais. In: Nardozza Jr A, Zerati Filho M, Borges dos Reis R (eds.) *Urologia Fundamental*. Plamark, Sao Paulo, 2010, pp. 383–389.

64. Wiser A, Raviv G, Weissenberg R, et al. Does age at orchidopexy impact on the results of testicular sperm extraction?. *Reprod Biomed Online* 2009;19(6):778–783.

65. Glina S, Vieira M. Prognostic factors for sperm retrieval in non-obstructive azoospermia. *Clinics* 2013;68(S1):121–124.

66. Walsh TJ, Wu AK, Croughan MS, Turek PJ. Differences in the clinical characteristics of primarily and secondarily infertile men with varicocele. *Fertil Steril* 2009;91:826–830.

67. Esteves SC, Glina S. Recovery of spermatogenesis after microsurgical subinguinal varicocele repair in azoospermic men based on testicular histology. *Int Braz J Urol* 2005;31:541–548.

68. Matthews GJ, Matthews ED, Goldstein M. Induction of spermatogenesis and achievement of pregnancy after microsurgical varicocelectomy in men with

azoospermia and severe oligoasthenospermia. *Fertil Steril* 1998;70(1):71–75.

69. Inci K, Hascicek M, Kara O, et al. Sperm retrieval and intracytoplasmic sperm injection in men with nonobstructive azoospermia, and treated and untreated varicocele. *J Urology* 2009;182(4):1500–1504.

70. Schlegel PN, Kaufmann J. Role of varicocelectomy in men with nonobstructive azoospermia. *Fertil Steril* 2004;81(6):1585–1588.

71. Berookhim BM, Palermo GD, Zaninovic N, Rosenwaks Z, Schlegel PN. Microdissection testicular sperm extraction in men with Sertoli cell–only testicular histology. *Fertil Steril* 2014;102:1282–1286.

72. Devroey P, Liu J, Nagy Z, et al. Pregnancies after testicular sperm extraction and intracytoplasmic sperm injection in non-obstructive azoospermia. *Hum Reprod* 1995;10(6):1457–1460.

73. Tsujimura A, Matsumiya K, Miyagawa Y, et al. Prediction of successful outcome of microdissection testicular sperm extraction in men with idiopathic nonobstructive azoospermia. *J Urol* 2004;172(5 Pt 1):1944–1947.

74. Marconi M, Keudel A, Diemer T, et al. Combined trifocal and microsurgical testicular sperm extraction is the best technique for testicular sperm retrieval in "low-chance" nonobstructive azoospermia. *Eur Urol* 2012;62:713.

75. Bromage SJ, Falconer DA, Lieberman BA, et al. Sperm retrieval rates in subgroups of primary azoospermic males. *Eur Urol* 2007;51:534.

76. Ziaee SA, Ezzatnegad M, Nowroozi M, et al. Prediction of successful sperm retrieval in patients with nonobstructive azoospermia. *Urol J* 2006;3:92.

77. Ezeh UI, Moore HD, Cooke ID. A prospective study of multiple needle biopsies versus a single open biopsy for testicular sperm extraction in men with non-obstructive azoospermia. *Hum Reprod* 1998;13:3075–3080.

78. Jarvi K, Lo K, Fischer A, et al. CUA Guideline: the workup of azoospermic males. *Can Urol Assoc J* 2010;4:163–167.

79. Deffieux X, Antoine JM. Inhibins, activins and anti-Mullerian hormone: structure, signalling pathways, roles and predictive value in reproductive medicine. *Gynecol Obstet Fertil* 2003;31(11):900–911.

80. Mitchell V, Boitrelle F, Pigny P, et al. Seminal plasma levels of anti-Mullerian hormone and inhibin B are not predictive of testicular sperm retrieval in nonobstructive azoospermia: a study of 139 men. *Fertil Steril* 2010;94(6):2147–2150.

81. Blagosklonova O, Fellmann F, Clavequin MC, Roux C, Bresson JL. AZFa deletions in Sertoli cell-only syndrome: a retrospective study. *Mol Hum Reprod* 2000;6:795–799.

82. Gonçalves C, Cunha M, Rocha E, et al. Y-chromosome microdeletions in nonobstructive azoospermia and severe oligozoospermia. *Asian J Androl* 2017;19(3):338–345

83. Miyaoka R, Orosz JE, Achermann AP, Esteves SC. Methods of surgical sperm extraction and implications for assisted reproductive technology success. *Panminerva Med* 2019;61(2):164–177.

84. Deruyver Y, Vanderschueren D, Van der Aa F. Outcome of microdissection TESE compared with conventional TESE in non-obstructive azoospermia: a systematic review. *Andrology* 2014;2:20–24.

85. Yukselten Y, Aydos OSE, Sunguroglu A, Aydos K.

Investigation of CD133 and CD24 as candidate azoospermia markers and their relationship with spermatogenesis defects. *Gene* 2019;706:211–221.

86. Aydos OS, Yukselten Y, Ozkavukcu S, Sunguroglu A, Aydos K. ADAMTS1 and ADAMTS5 metalloproteases produced by Sertoli cells: a potential diagnostic marker in azoospermia. *Syst Biol Reprod Med* 2019;65(1): 29–38.

87. Cao C, Wen Y, Wang X, et al. Testicular piRNA profile comparison between successful and unsuccessful micro-TESE retrieval in NOA patients. *J Assist Reprod Genet* 2018;35 (5):801–808.

Chapter 10

Methods for Enhancing Surgical Sperm Retrieval Success

Jordan A. Cohen and Ranjith Ramasamy

10.1 Introduction

Sperm retrieval techniques have been developed to obtain spermatozoa from the epididymis and testicles of azoospermic men. Following sperm acquisition, intracytoplasmic sperm injection (ICSI) may be used for couples interested in biological offspring when the male partner has azoospermia, or the sperm may be cryopreserved for future sperm injections. The surgical method of choice varies based on whether the azoospermia is secondary to obstructive or nonobstructive etiologies, both of which may be a result of congenital or acquired conditions. For patients with obstructive azoospermia, microsurgical ductal recanalization is highly successful; however, certain congenital anomalies or post-infectious etiologies may not offer a successful outcome and therefore sperm retrieval will be necessary. In this situation, successful spermatozoa retrieval can still be achieved from the epididymis or testicles, with the choice of sperm retrieval method based on the surgeon's preference and experience, and the patient's underlying etiology [1,2]. Patient preferences and female infertility can also play a role in recommending sperm retrieval in cases of obstructive azoospermia.

In men with obstructive azoospermia, percutaneous epididymal sperm aspiration (PESA) and microsurgical epididymal sperm aspiration (MESA) are two procedures that have been successfully utilized. Other notable techniques are percutaneous testicular sperm aspiration (TESA) and testicular sperm extraction (TESE) for failed epididymal retrieval in obstructive cases. There are clear advantages and disadvantages between the PESA and MESA techniques for obstructive cases. The PESA technique requires local anesthesia only, can generally be performed at shorter notice, requires no special equipment, and is 2–3 times cheaper than other methods such as MESA. However, a lower quantity of sperm is normally retrieved or there is a higher failure rate, with the

need to convert to TESE. The MESA technique requires an operating microscope, general anesthesia, and microsurgical training, but leads to higher sperm retrieval rates [3]. A study of 100 cases between these methods showed that PESA was successful in extraction 61 percent of the time. Upon PESA failure, MESA was subsequently performed, with a sperm retrieval rate of over 90 percent [4]. The technique selected is dependent on many factors, including cost, technology available, and overall knowledge of the procedure.

Nonobstructive azoospermia (NOA), the most common cause of azoospermia, is a result of spermatogenic failure that can be due to Sertoli-cell-only syndrome (SCOS), maturation arrest, or hypospermatogenesis. Patients with NOA were once considered to be infertile, with few treatment options secondary to the absence of sperm in the ejaculate. However, over the last two decades, a number of sperm retrieval techniques have revolutionized the treatment for NOA men. Primary therapies for patients with NOA are TESA and TESE. Again, each of these techniques has advantages and disadvantages related to ease, cost, repeatability, patient discomfort, risk of hematoma, and number of sperm retrieved for cryopreservation. Overall, success retrieval rates for patients with NOA, implying focal areas of sperm production within the testes, range from 30 to 60 percent; notably, sperm retrieval is the highest for micro-TESE, discussed subsequently, and the lowest for TESA [5,6].

10.2 Procedural Technique Enhancements

In the past decade, there has been a strong focus on newer techniques to achieve a more adequate number of, and the highest quality, sperm possible, while also preserving testicular function and reducing the number of repeated retrieval attempts. The microdissection technique was originally described in 1999 following observations noted during TESE procedures. To avoid damage to the testicular blood supply, the operating microscope was used to identify subtunical vessels prior to surgical incision at the time of biopsy. Microdissection has allowed for better visualization of seminiferous tubules to locate ones that are more promising. This technique, known as microdissection testicular sperm extraction (micro-TESE), is now considered the gold standard method of sperm retrieval utilized in patients suffering from NOA. A meta-analysis comprising 15 individual studies and 1890 patients compared the outcome differences between conventional TESE (cTESE) and micro-TESE. It was observed that spermatozoa retrieval for cTESE was successful in 35 percent of patients, while for micro-TESE, the success rate improved to 52 percent. In fact, microdissection has enhanced sperm retrieval success by making it 1.5 times more likely [7,8]. Moreover, targeting the larger tubules during microdissection at $15-20\times$ power also improves sperm retrieval yield and limits the amount of tissue that needs to be removed. If, however, microdissection fails, other techniques have shown some promise. One of these techniques is testicular mapping with fine-needle aspiration (FNA). These maps are performed on azoospermic men through simple and compound mapping techniques. In a series of 159 mapped cases, if at least one site was discovered containing mature sperm, this FNA map-guided TESE proved to be highly efficacious and rescued over 80 percent of those with prior failed micro-TESE attempts, resulting in successful retrieval [9].

10.3 Medical Adjuvant Therapy

Aside from FNA mapping, there are also various medical adjuvant therapies that have been shown to increase the success rates of micro-TESE by aiding spermatogenesis. Shiraishi et al. studied 48 men with NOA who had unsuccessful sperm retrieval results on first micro-TESE. Of these, 20 were not treated with any hormonal therapy, while 28 received daily injections for four months of human chorionic gonadotropin (hCG), and recombinant follicle-stimulating hormone (FSH) if endogenous gonadotropin levels decreased during hCG stimulation. A second micro-TESE procedure 4–5 months later was successful for more than 20 percent of the treated group, while no sperm was extracted from the control set [10].

Additionally, Hussein et al. have made a similar case for treatment with clomiphene citrate, a selective estrogen receptor modulator (SERM). A comparison of men with NOA was set up consisting of 116 patients who received no medical treatment and 442 who were administered clomiphene citrate in titrated doses. Micro-TESE was then subsequently performed in both groups. Overall, successful sperm retrieval was significantly higher for the clomiphene treated group (57 percent) than for the control group (33 percent) [11]. These findings indicate that surgeons can consider medical adjuvant therapy as a way to increase successful sperm extraction.

10.4 Innovations in Imaging

Despite all of these procedural improvements, it has remained a challenge to distinguish between seminiferous tubules with normal versus abnormal spermatogenesis. Recently, advances in high-level imaging of the seminiferous tubules has proven to be very promising; however, many of these are either in animal studies or only in preliminary testing stages and further work is required to optimize these techniques for human fertility issues. One technique that can possibly identify the presence of sperm within the tubules, without the need for tissue extraction, is multiphoton microscopy (MPM). In a mouse model, MPM has been shown to distinguish underlying microstructures of different seminiferous tubules. It works by using a low-energy infrared pulse laser to excite molecules, causing autofluorescence. However, MPM laser-guided techniques still need to be evaluated for long-term safety as lasers can potentially induce genetic abnormalities in gametes associated with ICSI [12]. A second technique for better visualization of spermatogenesis in tubules is full-field optical coherence tomography (FFOCT). This is a technique that uses white-light inference microscopy to produce high-resolution images. In a mouse model, FFOCT has been demonstrated to successfully image the tubules and determine the status of spermatogenesis [13]. While this technique holds promise for reducing the number of biopsies performed and decreasing operative time for the micro-TESE procedure, one limitation is its limited depth of imaging. Raman spectroscopy, a tool of laser-based optics, has successfully distinguished between those with Sertoli-cell-only histology and tubules with spermatogenesis. Finally, antibody labeling of sperm in the seminiferous tubules may reduce operative time and more readily identify sperm-filled tubules; however, the practicality of performing this in humans has not been proven [14]. Thus, in recent years, many innovative techniques such as microdissection and FNA mapping have come to clinical fruition. Additionally, enhanced imaging modalities, while in their infancy, are showing promise and likely will have a significant impact in the future. Together, these have significantly improved sperm retrieval success for those suffering from NOA. Large-scale collaborative studies will help identify the most promising imaging and retrieval technique combinations in this field.

10.5 Varicocele Repair and Sperm Retrieval

The last topic to be addressed in terms of improving sperm retrieval success and enhancing fertility is that of varicocele repair, especially for men with hypogonadism. Varicoceles can be associated with testicular dysfunction, testicular atrophy, and even azoospermia in some men. The etiology and pathophysiology of a varicocele is complex and multifactorial. Varicoceles not only reduce the quantity of Leydig cells, but qualitatively impair Leydig cell function, resulting in reduced serum testosterone levels and testicular volume loss compared to control subjects [15]. The exact mechanism by which a varicocele leads to impaired testicular function is unknown but likely relates to either altered testicular blood flow, increased scrotal temperatures, or redox imbalance. In a histologic study, Abdelrahim et al. evaluated bilateral testicular biopsies from 30 infertile men with varicocele taken both during varicocelectomies and postoperatively. Compared to healthy control subjects, preoperative biopsies showed reduced spermatogenesis with maturation arrest, dead spermatogenic epithelium, and a decrease in the volume of Leydig cells. After treatment, spermatogenesis improved in 22 (73 percent) of the patients. These patients also exhibited regeneration of the epithelium with the quantity of Leydig cells normalized in 18 patients (60 percent) [16]. Thus, improvement in serum testosterone levels following varicocele repair appears to be associated with improvements at the microstructural level.

Given that the presence of a palpable varicocele has a progressive and deleterious effect on spermatogenesis and testosterone production, there is growing evidence that early repair of varicoceles may prevent future infertility and androgen deficiency. About 30 percent of men with varicoceles have negatively impacted fertility likelihoods [17]. A Cochrane review in 2012 analyzed data from over 900 men in 10 different studies and found improvement in spontaneous pregnancy rates after varicocele repair from 26 to 40 percent [18]. Moreover, in the past few years, a strong relationship has been found between testicular sperm extraction techniques and varicocelectomy. Zampieri et al. conducted a study including men with both a clinical diagnosis of NOA and a unilateral grade three varicocele. Nineteen patients (group 1) underwent varicocelectomy three months before micro-TESE. The 16 patients of group 2 underwent varicocelectomy at the same time as the micro-TESE. Subsequently, the percentage of sperm retrieval during TESE was greater in group 1 (57.8 percent) than in group 2 (27 percent) [19]. These results highlight that varicocele repair significantly increases success rates of surgical sperm retrieval in patients with varicoceles. Thus, patients with hypogonadism and a varicocele should be counseled on the potential positive role of a varicocelectomy in improving fertility and similarly sperm retrieval.

10.6 Final Note

Overall, surgical sperm retrieval is becoming a more successful option for men with NOA or for select obstructive cases, which can later be used for ICSI or cryopreserved for the future. These developments, such as microsurgical techniques and better imaging modalities, including multiphoton microscopy and FFOCT, have successfully improved chances of sperm isolation. Finally, varicocele repair has proven to be significant prior to surgical sperm retrieval attempts as well.

References

1. Rosenlund B, Westlander G, Wood M, et al. Sperm retrieval and fertilization in repeated percutaneous epididymal sperm aspiration. *Hum Reprod Update* 1998;13(1O): 2805–2807.

2. Esteves SC, Lee W, Benjamin DJ, et al. Reproductive potential of men with obstructive azoospermia undergoing percutaneous sperm retrieval and intracytoplasmic sperm injection according to the cause of obstruction. *J Urology* 2013;189(1):232–237.

3. Coward R, Mills J. A step-by-step guide to office-based sperm retrieval for obstructive azoospermia. *Transl Androl Urol* 2017;6(4):730–744.

4. Lin YM, Hsu CC, Kuo TC, et al. Percutaneous epididymal sperm aspiration versus microsurgical

epididymal sperm aspiration for irreparable obstructive azoospermia: experience with 100 cases. *JFMA* 2000;99(6):459–465.

5. Esteves SC, Miyaoka R, Orosz JE, et al. An update on sperm retrieval for azoospermic males. *Clinics* 2013;68(S1):99–110.

6. Donoso P. Which is the best sperm retrieval technique for non-obstructive azoospermia? A systematic review. *Hum Reprod Update* 2007;13(6):539–549.

7. Ramasamy R, Yagan N, Schlegel PN. Structural and functional changes to the testis after conventional vs. microdissection testicular sperm extraction. *Urology* 2005;65:1190–1194.

8. Fraietta, R. Microdissection is the best way to perform sperm retrieval in men with non-obstructive azoospermia. *Int Braz J Urol* 2018;44(6):1063–1066.

9. Shin DH, Turek PJ. Sperm retrieval techniques. *Urol Nat Rev* 2013;10:723–730.

10. Shiraishi K, Ohmi C, Shimabukuro T, Matsuyama H. Human chorionic gonadotropin treatment prior to microdissection testicular sperm extraction in non-obstructive azoospermia. *Hum Reprod* 2012;27(2):331–339.

11. Hussein A, Ozgok Y, Ross L, Rao P, Niederberger C. Optimization of spermatogenesis-regulating hormones in patients with non-obstructive azoospermia and its impact on sperm retrieval. *BJU Int* 2013;111(3):110–114.

12. Ramasamy R, Sterling J, Fisher ES, et al. Identification of spermatogenesis with multiphoton microscopy: an evaluation in a rodent model. *J Urol* 2011;186:2487–2492.

13. Ramasamy R, Sterling J, Manzoor M, et al. Full field optical coherence tomography can identify spermatogenesis in a rodent Sertoli-cell only model. *J Pathol Inform* 2012;3:4.

14. Ran R, Kohn TP, Ramasamy R. Innovations in surgical management of nonobstructive azoospermia. *Indian J Urol* 2016;32(1):15–20.

15. Guercio C, Patil D, Mehta A. Hypogonadism is independently associated with varicocele repair in a contemporary cohort of men in the USA. *Asian J Androl* 2018;21(1):45–49.

16. Abdelrahim F, Mostafa A, Hamdy A, et al. Testicular morphology and function in varicocele patients: pre-operative and post-operative histopathology. *Br J Urol* 1993;72:643–647.

17. Agarwal A, Deepinder F, Cocuzza M, et al. Efficacy of varicocelectomy in improving semen parameters: new meta-analytical approach. *Urology.* 2007;70(3):532–538.

18. Kroese AC, de Lange NM, Collins J, Evers JL. Surgery or embolization for varicoceles in subfertile men. *Cochrane Database Syst Rev* 2012;10: CD000479.

19. Zampieri N, Bosaro L, Costantini C, Zaffagnini S, Zampieri G. Relationship between testicular sperm extraction and varicocelectomy in patients with varicocele and nonobstructive azoospermia. *Urology* 2013; 82(1):74–77.

Critical Factors for Optimizing Sperm Handling and ICSI Outcomes

Edson Borges Jr., Amanda Souza Setti, and Daniela Paes de Almeida Ferreira Braga

11.1 Introduction

In 1992, a major development in the field of male infertility and assisted reproduction, intracytoplasmic sperm injection (ICSI), was introduced. However, it was only a few years later that the successful use of sperm retrieved directly from epididymis and testes was reported for the treatment of male infertility by virtue of azoospermia.

Azoospermia, observed in 1 percent of the general population and in 10–15 percent of infertile men, is the absence of sperm in the ejaculate after assessment of at least two centrifuged semen samples, and is clinically categorized as obstructive azoospermia (OA) or nonobstructive azoospermia (NOA) [1].

Successful sperm retrieval is possible in practically 100 percent of patients with OA and in 50 percent of patients with NOA using the following techniques that capture spermatozoa directly from the epididymis and testes: percutaneous epididymal sperm aspiration (PESA), microsurgical epididymal sperm aspiration (MESA), testicular sperm aspiration (TESA), testicular sperm extraction (TESE), and microdissection testicular sperm extraction (micro-TESE) [2]. Despite the fertilization rate being higher with epididymal sperm, similar clinical pregnancy and implantation rates are obtained with testicular or epididymal spermatozoa, regardless of whether the azoospermia is obstructive or nonobstructive [3]. Also, there is evidence that the success of the first TESA procedure predicts the results of additional attempts in NOA patients [4].

This chapter summarizes the development of the processing and selection of surgically retrieved sperm, as well as the use of oocyte activation in couples with azoospermia.

11.2 Timing of Sperm Retrieval

Sperm harvesting can be performed prior to or in conjunction with oocyte retrieval from the female partner. There are advantages and disadvantages associated with both method schedules; ultimately, the decision is made according to the assisted fertilization center's preference.

Despite the difficulties in scheduling sperm retrieval in conjunction with oocyte retrieval, most of the centers prefer to handle fresh sperm samples rather than frozen. Thus, sperm harvesting is performed the day of egg retrieval, mainly in male partners with known OA, in which sperm retrieval is supposed to be a simple procedure.

Nevertheless, harvesting sperm prior to oocyte retrieval obviates several concerns related to the center's availability of operating and recovery rooms, surgeons, and embryologists in the busy morning hours. Moreover, it has to be considered that, in many cases, the oocyte retrieval day is not on the date originally scheduled. Both epididymal and testicular sperm are able to survive for up to 72 hours if properly incubated in culture media. In fact, sperm extracted directly from the tubules of the testicular tissue may take a while to become motile. In addition, sperm motility can be induced with a motility enhancer for the selection of viable sperm for ICSI.

When the odds of finding sperm are low, there is always the option of harvesting and freezing sperm in advance. If no sperm is retrieved, the couple has to choose between using donor sperm or freezing the entire cohort of retrieved oocytes until another sperm retrieval technique can be scheduled. Similar ICSI outcomes are yielded when freeze–thawed or fresh, testicular or epididymal spermatozoa are used, particularly when high numbers of spermatozoa are harvested [5].

Whenever micro-TESE is indicated, it is usually performed the day before oocyte retrieval due to the complexity of the procedure [6]. It is important to mention that some couples may be reluctant to undergo surgery together because of personal reasons, such as lack of home assistance and transportation, among others.

11.3 Processing of Surgically Retrieved Sperm for ICSI

Epididymal aspirates, such as MESA and PESA, are generally mixed with buffered culture medium before an aliquot is used for count, motility, and morphology analysis. Aspirates containing low sperm count can be processed by double washing and centrifugation, while those with high sperm count can be treated with density gradient centrifugation followed by double washing [reviewed in 7]. An aliquot of the processed sample is placed on a Petri dish and covered with oil until the moment of ICSI. Supernumerary sperm can be frozen and used in subsequent ICSI cycles.

Sperm aspirated directly from the testis are poured in a dry tube or in culture medium droplets under oil until sperm selection for ICSI. For sperm retrieved through TESE specimens, different processing has been described, such as mechanical processing, and the use of enzymes or erythrocyte-lysing buffer to improve sperm recovery. A method of mechanical testicular tissue homogenization using a loose-fitting glass pestle, followed by repeated aspiration through a 16 G needle, has been proposed by Oates et al. [8].

One study compared four mechanical methods to retrieve testicular spermatozoa – rough shredding, fine mincing, vortexing, and crushing in a grinder with pestle – and demonstrated that the most effective method regarding motile sperm count and morphology was fine mincing [9]. In fact, rupture of seminiferous tubules by shredding and fine mincing is the most used testicular tissue processing method. The testicular tissue is placed in a Petri dish containing buffered culture medium and shredded with needles, microscope slides, or scissors, thus releasing sperm into the medium. The sample is assessed under an inverted microscope or a phase-contrast microscope. Upon the easy identification of sperm, the sample is allowed to rest for the sedimentation of the remaining tissue pieces, and then the supernatant is centrifuged, removed, and resuspended. The sample is smeared on a Petri dish overlaid with oil, from which the sperm will be selected from ICSI.

Red blood cell contamination in the testicular tissue sample is a recurrent feature that may hinder the identification of spermatozoa. In those cases, the tissue sample may be exposed to an erythrocyte-lysing buffer (ELB) after shredding. This method improves sperm recovery and selection, and reduces the sperm identification interval [10].

In men presenting with limited sperm production, mechanical sperm extraction can be complicated and time-consuming, and thus testicular sperm can be extracted enzymatically to improve sperm recovery. The most common enzymes used to digest testicular tissue are type IA and IV collagenases. The collagenases are able to digest the collagen present in the membranes and extracellular matrix. It has been demonstrated that the use of collagenase results in the recovery of sperm in nearly 26 percent of men undergoing ICSI, after no sperm had been found post-mechanical shredding [10]. Therefore, enzymatic digestion is routinely used after failure of sperm identification with mechanical shredding. Even though the effectiveness of the enzymatic methods on testicular sperm recovery has already been proven, the mechanical approaches are more widespread and routinely applied.

There are still several challenges hindering the management of infertility in men with NOA. Clinically, there is a need to develop diagnostic tests for the prediction of successful testicular sperm retrieval. At the laboratory level, some methods have already been developed to enhance sperm selection in those patients.

11.4 Selection of Surgically Retrieved Sperm for ICSI

Successful retrieval of sperm is only the first step toward the achievement of successful ICSI outcomes. In fact, ICSI performed with ejaculated sperm already made us wonder about the potential impact of the non-natural sperm selection that is performed by the embryologist. This question is even more pressing when testicular sperm is used for ICSI. Therefore, methods to aid in the selection of not only the "best-looking," but also the most functional sperm are in order.

Extended culture of surgically retrieved spermatozoa may allow sperm maturation and attainment of motility; thus, several centers opt to perform sperm retrieval on the day before oocyte collection, and incubate the sperm sample until ICSI is performed. These improvements have been demonstrated in men with OA and NOA. It is noteworthy that sperm improvements peaked within 48 hours of culture, and intervals higher than two days were associated

91

with sperm aging, represented by higher DNA damage and chromosomal abnormalities [11].

Nevertheless, even after extended culture of surgically retrieved sperm, some samples fail to provide motile sperm for ICSI. In those cases, the use of adjunct sperm selection techniques is recommended [reviewed in 7].

11.4.1 Mechanical Touch Technique

The mechanical touch technique, initially described as the sperm tail flexibility test, has been applied for the identification of immotile sperm viability prior to ICSI. It relies on the fact that immotile vital and non-vital sperm differ in tail flexibility when touched with the microinjection pipette, in which vital sperm are flexible and non-vital sperm are rigid. In the presence of tail flexibility, the sperm head will not move along with the tail, and the tail will return to its original positioning. Conversely, the sperm head will move together with a rigid tail when touched with the pipette, and the tail will not recover initial positioning.

Studies have demonstrated similar rates of fertilization, pregnancy, and delivery when motile testicular sperm and immotile testicular sperm selected with this technique were used for ICSI [12]. The advantages of the mechanical touch technique are that it is performed in real time, and it is free of dyes and chemicals; thus, it allows the analyzed sperm to be used for ICSI. In contrast, inter- and intra-observer variability may occur as a result of the subjectivity of the test, and it may be time-consuming to touch sperm by sperm before injection.

11.4.2 Hypoosmotic Swelling Test

The hypoosmotic swelling test evaluates the functional integrity of the plasma membrane, demonstrated by the capacity of the sperm to react to hypoosmotic media. Live sperm cells presumably possess intact and functional membranes, and will present tail swelling or curling due to water influx when exposed to hypotonic media, while dead sperm with disintegrated membranes will not react [7].

11.4.3 Chemical Motility Enhancers

Pentoxifylline and theophylline are methylxanthine derivatives used for treating vascular disorders due to their hemorrheological property. They are also phosphodiesterase inhibitors that can increase the levels of cyclic adenosine monophosphate, which plays a role in sperm motility. Pentoxifylline was introduced into the clinical routine of IVF centers in 1988; it took a decade to demonstrate its effects on immotile testicular sperm. The addition of pentoxifylline to sperm retrieved from the epididymis or testis resulted in motility gain and successful ICSI outcomes. The effects of theophylline on sibling oocytes were later investigated and the enhancement of sperm motility was confirmed.

Despite the sperm being washed post-methylxanthine treatment, the toxicity of these chemical compounds has been questioned. Nevertheless, so far, there is no evidence of abnormalities in the offspring, and thus the addition of methylxanthines may significantly reduce the time for sperm identification and selection, with no apparent detriment to the outcomes of pregnancy [7,13].

11.4.4 Laser-Assisted Immotile Sperm Selection

Laser-assisted immotile sperm selection (LAISS) was introduced in 2004 by Aktan et al. [14] and discriminates between viable and nonviable (dead) immotile sperm by assessing tail curling, as detected in live sperm when hit by a single laser shot close to the end of the tail. In contrast, the lack of tail dislocation demonstrates that the sperm is dead. This is a safe, chemical-free, and rapid sperm selection technique that provides an immediate response regarding sperm viability. Recently, testicular sperm selected via this technique demonstrated increased fertilization potential [15]. The main obstacle to its widespread application is the high cost of the equipment.

11.4.5 Birefringence: Polarization Microscopy

Pioneered by Baccetti [16], the analysis of birefringence (double reflection) in sperm cells, as confirmed by transmission electron microscopy, is an indicator of structural normality. The presence of birefringence suggests an organized and compact structure that reflects normal sperm nuclei, acrosomes, and flagella, whereas non-vital sperm lack birefringence because of their diverse texture. Therefore, the use of polarization microscopy for sperm selection prior to ICSI was proposed based on the properties of birefringence that human spermatozoon naturally possesses. The sperm selection via sperm head birefringence was demonstrated to be of benefit for oligoasthenoteratozoospermic samples and for testicular-retrieved sperm [17]. Nevertheless, the scientific literature concerning the efficacy of sperm selection using polarization microscopy is controversial [reviewed in 18], and reliable cut-off values are still needed. In addition, as polarization microscopy is an expensive asset to the IVF laboratory, cheaper sperm selection methods are available, thus hindering more widespread application of this technique.

11.5 Artificial Oocyte Activation

Sperm and egg interaction involves a series of physiological and biochemical events, involving species recognition, adhesion, and then fusion between gametes. The ultimate step, oocyte activation, is the starting point of a developmental program leading to the formation of a new individual [19]. Oocyte activation involves a characteristic pattern of intracellular calcium (Ca^{2+}) oscillations, which orchestrate a series of further key events, such as cortical granule material exocytosis, prevention of polyspermy, polar body extrusion, cytoskeletal rearrangements, resumption of meiosis, formation of pronuclei, initiation of the first mitotic division in the new zygote, recruitment of maternal mRNA, and regulation of gene expression [20].

The exact mechanism responsible for oocyte activation has been a matter of debate for decades. Accumulating evidence has suggested that a catalytic substance, present in the sperm head, initiated Ca^{2+} release in the ooplasm following gamete fusion and the PLCζ (1-phosphatidylinositol 4,5-bisphosphate phosphodiesterase zeta-1) has been indicated as the key sperm oocyte activation factor [21].

It has been postulated that fertile men present a significantly higher proportion of sperm exhibiting PLCζ than infertile men. Reduced levels, abnormal localization, reduced activity/expression or genetic mutations in PLCζ have been associated with oocyte activation deficiency and therefore ICSI failure [22], even in patients with normal sperm parameters [23].

It has been reported that up to 70 percent of unfertilized, metaphase II oocytes after ICSI contain a swollen sperm head, indicating that the oocyte may have been correctly injected but failed to become activated to complete the second meiotic division [24].

Intracytoplasmic sperm injection was introduced to overcome severe male infertility, and although the procedure results in an average fertilization rate of 70 percent, in rare cases fertilization fails due to the lack of oocyte activation. Total fertilization failure occurs in 2–3 percent of ICSI cycles.

Oocyte activation failure can be compensated by artificially increasing calcium in the oocyte, the so-called artificial oocyte activation (AOA). Protocols used for AOA can be classified based on whether the mechanism evoking the Ca^{2+} trigger that promotes fertilization is mechanical, electrical, or chemical. However, one should keep in mind that ICSI AOA is not beneficial for patients with a suspected oocyte-related activation deficiency. Artificial oocyte activation is still an experimental technique and should be carefully considered.

11.5.1 Mechanical Activation

Mechanical oocyte activation entails a modified ICSI technique, in which the microinjection pipette is advanced during the ICSI procedure and peripheral cytoplasm is aspirated. Subsequently, the aspirated cytoplasm and the spermatozoon are deposited into the center of the oocyte.

Tesarik et al. [25] reported an ICSI technique primarily based on the repeated dislocation of the central ooplasm to the periphery, which increases the intracellular concentration of free Ca^{2+} either by creating an influx of Ca^{2+} or by the release of stored Ca^{2+} from cell organelles. It was suggested that this mechanical oocyte activation may have an immediate clinical application in patients with repeated fertilization failures, after ICSI, suspected to be caused by insufficiency of PLCζ or by a defective oocyte response to this sperm factor [25]. This technique may represent an alternative to the use of Ca^{2+} ionophores. The possibility of using a simple modification of the standard ICSI micromanipulation technique instead of ionophores alleviates concerns about the possible harmful effects on human embryos.

Considering a possible negative effect of this rather vigorous injection technique on further preimplantation development, Ebner et al. [26] developed a modified ICSI technique based on the hypothetical accumulation of highly polarized mitochondria. The cytoplasm in the periphery of the oocyte is thought to be rich in

93

mitochondria with high inner-membrane potential and high metabolic ATP activity. Therefore, this method aims to accumulate peripheral mitochondria and thus increase energy sources at the site of subsequent pronuclear formation [26]. The authors suggested that the modified ICSI possibly accumulates mitochondria with a higher inner mitochondrial membrane potential and may be a reliable and safe alternative to conventional ICSI leading to comparable rates of blastocyst formation, implantation, and clinical pregnancy. In particular, this technology was proven to be useful in cases of previous failure of fertilization in ICSI cycles [26].

11.5.2 Electrical Activation

An electrical field can generate micropores in the cell membrane of gametes to induce sufficient Ca^{2+} influx through the pores to activate cytoplasm through a Ca^{2+}-dependent mechanism. In animal models, oocytes injected with secondary spermatocytes or spermatids were fertilized when stimulated by electroporation and developed into normal offspring when the resultant embryos were transferred to a recipient uterus [27].

Yanagida et al. were the first to use ICSI followed by electrical oocyte activation for human oocyte activation, which resulted in healthy twins for a couple with previously failed fertilization after ICSI [28]. This study was followed by others with different experimental designs and different situations (i.e., previous fertilization failure, severe oligoasthenozoospermia, or NOA with total teratozoospermia).

Mansour et al. [29] evaluated the electroactivation of oocytes after ICSI in 241 cycles with either severe oligoasthenoteratozoospermia or azoospermia. For this trial, sibling oocytes for each patient were randomly divided after ICSI into two groups: the study group (electroactivation) and the control group (without electroactivation). Electrical activation resulted in a significant improvement in the fertilization rate after ICSI.

Oocyte electrical activation was also assessed in infertile couples having a history of total fertilization failure in previous ICSI cycles. For this study, a significantly increased fertilization rate and high-quality embryos rate was noted [30].

Some studies evaluated the effectiveness of oocyte electrical activation in non-fertilized oocytes after ICSI (rescue oocytes activation). Traditionally oocyte electrical activation is performed, on average, 30 min after ICSI. For the rescue oocyte activation, oocytes showing no evidence of fertilization by 16–24 hours after ICSI are electroactivated.

Zhang et al. [31] demonstrated that electrical stimulation can "rescue" oocytes that fail to fertilize by 24 hours after ICSI and stimulate them to complete the second meiotic division, form pronuclei, and undergo early embryonic development. One hundred failed-to-fertilize oocytes after ICSI were randomly assigned by stratified allocation according to oocyte grading before ICSI. Fifty unfertilized oocytes were electroactivated and the remaining 50 unfertilized oocytes were treated in the same way but without electrical activation. The embryo formation rates in the electrically activated group were 80 percent compared to 16 percent in the control group, suggesting once again that failed-to-fertilize oocytes after ICSI seem to be able to resume embryonic development after electrical activation. However, the study failed to demonstrate whether such embryos are capable of implanting.

It has been demonstrated that electroactivation results in a rapid rise in Ca^{2+} inside the oocyte, which gradually decreases to the original level in about 300 s. The aforementioned studies suggested that the oocyte electrical activation soon after ICSI or in unfertilized oocytes may be a promising approach for the treatment of patients with the risk of fertilization failure or those with high fertilization failure rates in previous cycles. However, electrical oocyte activation has not yet been proven to be the most efficient and safe method for oocyte activation in humans. Moreover, there is insufficient evidence available from randomized controlled trials to judge the efficacy and safety of this method in couples undergoing assisted reproduction cycles, and long-term follow-up studies are needed to ensure safety.

11.5.3 Chemical Activation

The potential of Ca^{2+} ionophores to support AOA and yield high fertilization rates was shown at the beginning of the ICSI era [32]. Since that time, a number of studies have been conducted to assess the value of Ca^{2+} ionophores and others chemical agents as methods of AOA in humans. Chemical oocyte activation remained the most common method for AOA.

Chemical activation agents are classified based on the Ca^{2+} response they elicit in mammalian oocytes: (1) single Ca^{2+} transients, (2) dynamic Ca^{2+} oscillations, and (3) oocyte activation independent of the initial Ca^{2+} trigger

11.5.3.1 Agents Inducing Single Ca^{2+} Transients

Ca^{2+} Ionophores

Calcium ionophores, such as ionomycin and calcimycin, confer high permeability to cell membranes, allowing Ca^{2+} ions to penetrate through. Oocytes exposed to Ca^{2+} ionophores experience an increase of free intracytoplasmic Ca^{2+}, which results from Ca^{2+} influx, as well as Ca^{2+} release from the intracellular stores, particularly the endoplasmic reticulum.

When poor ICSI oocyte activation rates are observed, Ca^{2+} ionophores are the most commonly used treatment option. Ca^{2+} ionophores have been used in many cases of complete activation failure or previous high rates of fertilization failure.

The effect of AOA with a Ca^{2+} ionophore on ICSI cycles using surgically retrieved sperm has also been suggested. Borges et al. [33] demonstrated that AOA might be useful in improving ICSI outcomes in azoospermic patients when epididymal, but not testicular, fresh spermatozoa are injected [34]. It was also suggested that AOA may be a useful tool to improve ICSI outcomes when ejaculated or epididymal spermatozoa are used in younger, but not older, female partners [34]. These findings highlight the theory that both sperm maturity and oocyte quality play roles in oocyte activation.

A recently published meta-analysis suggested that the use of Ca^{2+} ionophores after ICSI treatment increases the overall pregnancy rate per embryo transfer and the live-birth rate per embryo transfer and treatment cycle [35]. It has also been demonstrated that the use of Ca^{2+} ionophores after ICSI increases the multiple pregnancy rate [35].

The results after analysis of secondary outcomes were also encouraging: the fertilization, cleavage, blastocyst formation, and implantation rates were all increased after the use of Ca^{2+} ionophores [35].

Although it can give rise to live births in cycles that would otherwise fail, Ca^{2+} ionophores can only cause one or, in some protocols, two large Ca^{2+} increases, which fails to mimic the multiple Ca^{2+} oscillations that occur at fertilization.

The importance of Ca^{2+} oscillation in embryo development and pregnancy outcome has been highlighted. In contrast, the aberrant induced calcium rise, which includes a single surge without subsequent oscillations, when chemical and electrical methods of AOA are used raises concerns regarding the safety and physiological relevance of AOA and requires further clinical evaluation.

Nevertheless, accumulating evidence supports the biosafety of ionomycin as an activating agent. First, high oocyte survival rates are observed following chemical AOA in mouse and human oocytes. Moreover, ionomycin did not increase the incidence of meiotic errors of maternal origin in human oocytes [36].

Most importantly, the follow-up studies of children born following AOA support the safety of this methodology [37,38]. Together, these data endorse the use of AOA for clinical applications. Defining a proper indication, however, requires further investigation. Diagnostic tools to identify cases that could benefit from AOA are needed to guide clinicians.

Nevertheless, the use of ionophores remains experimental. The knowledge concerning its potential cytotoxic, teratogenic, and mutagenic effects on embryos and offspring is still insufficient. No long-term follow-up studies of children born after chemical ICSI AOA are available yet.

11.5.3.2 Agents Inducing Oscillatory Ca^{2+} Signaling

Thimerosal

Thimerosal has the capacity to induce Ca^{2+} oscillations by oxidizing protein thiol groups at the inositol trisphosphate receptors. As a consequence, the receptors become sensitized to the cytosolic concentration of inositol trisphosphate, a key component determining intracellular Ca^{2+} oscillations and oocyte activation.

Strontium

Strontium (Sr^{2+}) is able to replace Ca^{2+} for triggering somatic cellular responses and eliciting calcium oscillations, not only a single surge like Ca^{2+} ionophores. Treatment with Sr^{2+} has been previously proposed as a strategy to "rescue" human oocytes that failed to fertilize after ICSI [39].

Even though Sr^{2+} is the most efficient method for mouse oocyte activation, leading to high blastocyst formation rates, its efficiency in activating human oocytes is still under debate [39,40].

95

Recombinant PLCζ

Accumulating evidence favors the idea that Ca^{2+} oscillations are triggered after entry of PLCζ into the oocyte cytoplasm. The activation of mammalian oocytes at fertilization involves an extensive series of Ca^{2+} oscillations.

Each Ca^{2+} spike lasts about 1 min, and the Ca^{2+} transients occur at intervals of 5–30 min. Artificial oocyte activation to overcome failed fertilization after ICSI in human oocytes typically employs Ca^{2+} ionophores to produce a single cytosolic Ca^{2+} increase. In contrast, recombinant PLCζ causes Ca^{2+} oscillations indistinguishable from those occurring during fertilization and subsequent development of embryos up to the blastocyst stage at rates similar to those seen after fertilization.

PLCζ remains the only physiological agent that has been repeatedly shown to produce a prolonged series of Ca^{2+} oscillations in all mammalian oocytes studied, including human oocytes [41,42]. In this regard, the use of PLCζ as an oocyte activation agent seems promising, particularly in cases where sperm is devoid of PLCζ, such as in globozoospermia or in patients carrying punctual mutations in the PLCζ gene.

Sanusi et al. [43] tested the efficacy of AOA with recombinant PLCζ in a scenario of ICSI fertilization failure. The authors compared PLCζ with other activation stimuli (Ca^{2+} ionophore or with Sr^{2+} media) in a mouse model of failed oocyte activation after ICSI. All tested treatments rescued oocyte activation, although Sr^{2+} and PLCζ gave the highest rates of development to blastocyst.

When recombinant PLCζ was given to oocytes previously injected with control sperm, they developed normally to the blastocyst stage at rates similar to that after control ICSI, suggesting that recombinant human PLCζ is an efficient means of rescuing oocyte activation after ICSI failure and that it can be effectively used even if the sperm already contains endogenous Ca^{2+} releasing activity.

11.5.3.3 Oocyte Activation Independent of the Initial Ca^{2+} Trigger

Puromycin

Puromycin is known to inhibit mitogen-activating protein kinase (MAPK), which is a component of cytostatic factor in mammals' oocytes. Mitogen-activating protein kinase possibly activates a positive regulator of the maturation promoting factor (MPF) or inhibits negative regulators. Therefore, puromycin may decrease MPF activity via suppression of MAPK, resulting in the formation of a pronucleus.

It has been reported that puromycin induces parthenogenetic activation in about 90 percent of human oocytes, and the combination of puromycin and a Ca^{2+} ionophore could effectively produce human and mouse haploid parthenogenones.

This combination has been tested for activating unfertilized oocytes after ICSI. It was demonstrated that Ca^{2+} ionophores with puromycin can stimulate unfertilized oocytes 20–68 h after ICSI to complete the second meiosis, to form pronuclei, and to undergo early embryonic development. Furthermore, nearly all embryos had a normal set of sex chromosomes and could develop normally. All of these findings suggest that the chemical approach has the potential to "rescue" unfertilized oocytes after ICSI [44].

11.6 Conclusion

Several tests for sperm selection of viable immotile spermatozoa exist, with particular advantages and disadvantages intrinsic to each one. The most appropriate method for sperm selection will depend on the expertise of the laboratory staff and available equipment. Despite the need for further studies to confirm the benefits of these methods for the improvement of ICSI outcomes, evidence is already available that points to higher fertilization and pregnancy rates in couples with a severe male factor infertility and/or testicular-retrieved spermatozoa. Therefore, the use of at least one of these methods of sperm selection should be incorporated into a modern IVF laboratory routine when dealing with immotile sperm.

Despite incorporating efficient sperm selection methods for ICSI, complete or nearly complete fertilization failure, after ICSI, may occur in up to 5 percent of ICSI cycles. Failure of oocyte activation is thought to be an important cause of fertilization failure following conventional ICSI, and AOA methods may overcome these limitations.

The efficiency of AOA has been proved in terms of increased pregnancy and live-birth rates; however, the literature lacks robust evidence concerning the long-term outcomes or whether gene expression is affected by AOA. Future studies should determine the long-term treatment safety of AOA so that it can be effectively included in clinical routines to avoid fertilization failures.

References

1. Male Infertility Best Practice Policy Committee of the American Urological Association Practice Committee of the American Society for Reproductive Medicine. Report on evaluation of the azoospermic male. *Fertil Steril* 2006;86: S210–S215.

2. Proctor M, Johnson N, van Peperstraten AM, Phillipson G. Techniques for surgical retrieval of sperm prior to intra-cytoplasmic sperm injection (ICSI) for azoospermia. *Cochrane Database Syst Rev* 2008;2: CD002807.

3. Semiao-Francisco L, Braga DP, Figueira Rde C, et al. Assisted reproductive technology outcomes in azoospermic men: 10 years of experience with surgical sperm retrieval. *Aging Male* 2010;13:44–50.

4. Borges E, Jr., Braga DP, Bonetti TC, Pasqualotto FF, Iaconelli A, Jr. Predictive factors of repeat sperm aspiration success. *Urology* 2010;75:87–91.

5. Urman B, Alatas C, Aksoy S, et al. Performing testicular or epididymal sperm retrieval prior to the injection of hCG. *J Assist Reprod Genet* 1998;15:125–128.

6. Levran D, Ginath S, Farhi J, et al. Timing of testicular sperm retrieval procedures and in vitro fertilization-intracytoplasmic sperm injection outcome. *Fertil Steril* 2001;76:380–383.

7. Verheyen G, Popovic-Todorovic B, Tournaye H. Processing and selection of surgically-retrieved sperm for ICSI: a review. *Basic Clin Androl* 2017;27:6.

8. Oates RD, Mulhall J, Burgess C, Cunningham D, Carson R. Fertilization and pregnancy using intentionally cryopreserved testicular tissue as the sperm source for intracytoplasmic sperm injection in 10 men with non-

obstructive azoospermia. *Hum Reprod* 1997;12:734–739.

9. Verheyen G, De Croo I, Tournaye H, et al. Comparison of four mechanical methods to retrieve spermatozoa from testicular tissue. *Hum Reprod* 1995;10:2956–2959.

10. Crabbé E, Verheyen G, Silber S, et al. Enzymatic digestion of testicular tissue may rescue the intracytoplasmic sperm injection cycle in some patients with non-obstructive azoospermia. *Hum Reprod* 1998;13:2791–2796.

11. Dalzell LH, McVicar CM, McClure N, Lutton D, Lewis SE. Effects of short and long incubations on DNA fragmentation of testicular sperm. *Fertil Steril* 2004;82:1443–1445.

12. de Oliveira NM, Vaca Sanchez R, Rodriguez Fiesta S, et al. Pregnancy with frozen-thawed and fresh testicular biopsy after motile and immotile sperm microinjection, using the mechanical touch technique to assess viability. *Hum Reprod* 2004;19:262–265.

13. Loughlin KR, Agarwal A. Use of theophylline to enhance sperm function. *Arch Androl* 1992;28:99–103.

14. Aktan TM, Montag M, Duman S, et al. Use of a laser to detect viable but immotile spermatozoa. *Andrologia* 2004;36:366–369.

15. Nordhoff V, Schuring AN, Krallmann C, et al. Optimizing TESE-ICSI by laser-assisted selection of immotile spermatozoa and polarization microscopy for selection of oocytes. *Andrology* 2013;1:67–74.

16. Baccetti B. Microscopical advances in assisted reproduction. *J Submicrosc Cytol Pathol* 2004;36:333–339.

17. Tournaye H, Verheyen G, Nagy P, et al. Are there any predictive factors for successful testicular sperm recovery in azoospermic

patients?. *Hum Reprod* 1997;12:80–86.

18. Henkel R. Novel sperm tests and their importance. In Agarwal A, Borges Jr. E, Setti A (eds.) *Non-Invasive Sperm Selection for In Vitro Fertilization*. Springer, New York, 2015, pp. 23–40.

19. Ciapa B,Chiri S. Egg activation: upstream of the fertilization calcium signal. *Biol Cell* 2000;92:215–233.

20. Malcuit C, Kurokawa M, Fissore RA. Calcium oscillations and mammalian egg activation. *J Cell Physiol* 2006;206:565–573.

21. Yeste M, Jones C, Amdani SN, Patel S, Coward K. Oocyte activation deficiency: a role for an oocyte contribution? *Hum Reprod Update* 2016;22:23–47.

22. Yelumalai S, Yeste M, Jones C, et al. Total levels, localization patterns, and proportions of sperm exhibiting phospholipase C zeta are significantly correlated with fertilization rates after intracytoplasmic sperm injection. *Fertil Steril* 2015;104:561–8 e4.

23. Lee HC, Arny M, Grow D, et al. Protein phospholipase C Zeta1 expression in patients with failed ICSI but with normal sperm parameters. *J Assist Reprod Genet* 2014;31:749–756.

24. Mahutte NG, Arici A. Failed fertilization: is it predictable? *Curr Opin Obstet Gynecol* 2003;15:211–218.

25. Tesarik J, Rienzi L, Ubaldi F, Mendoza C, Greco E. Use of a modified intracytoplasmic sperm injection technique to overcome sperm-borne and oocyte-borne oocyte activation failures. *Fertil Steril* 2002;78:619–624.

26. Ebner T, Moser M, Sommergruber M, Jesacher K, Tews G. Complete oocyte activation failure after ICSI can be overcome by a modified injection technique. *Hum Reprod* 2004;19:1837–1841.

27. Sasagawa I, Yanagimachi R. Comparison of methods for activating mouse oocytes for spermatid nucleus transfer. *Zygote* 1996;4:269–274.

28. Yanagida K, Katayose H, Yazawa H, et al. Successful fertilization and pregnancy following ICSI and electrical oocyte activation. *Hum Reprod* 1999;14:1307–1311.

29. Mansour R, Fahmy I, Tawab NA, et al. Electrical activation of oocytes after intracytoplasmic sperm injection: a controlled randomized study. *Fertil Steril* 2009;91:133–139.

30. Baltaci V, Ayvaz OU, Unsal E, et al. The effectiveness of intracytoplasmic sperm injection combined with piezoelectric stimulation in infertile couples with total fertilization failure. *Fertil Steril* 2010;94:900–904.

31. Zhang J, Wang CW, Blaszcyzk A, et al. Electrical activation and in vitro development of human oocytes that fail to fertilize after intracytoplasmic sperm injection. *Fertil Steril* 1999;72:509–512.

32. Tesarik J, Sousa M, Mendoza C. Sperm-induced calcium oscillations of human oocytes show distinct features in oocyte center and periphery. *Mol Reprod Dev* 1995;41:257–263.

33. Borges E, Jr., de Almeida Ferreira Braga DP, de Sousa Bonetti TC, Iaconelli A, Jr., Franco JG, Jr. Artificial oocyte activation with calcium ionophore A23187 in intracytoplasmic sperm injection cycles using surgically retrieved spermatozoa. *Fertil Steril* 2009;92:131–136.

34. Borges E, Jr., de Almeida Ferreira Braga DP, de Sousa Bonetti TC, Iaconelli A, Jr., Franco JG, Jr. Artificial oocyte activation using calcium ionophore in ICSI cycles with spermatozoa from different sources. *Reprod Biomed Online* 2009;18:45–52.

35. Murugesu S, Saso S, Jones BP, et al. Does the use of calcium ionophore during artificial oocyte activation demonstrate an effect on pregnancy rate? A meta-analysis. *Fertil Steril* 2017;108:468–482 e3.

36. Capalbo A, Ottolini CS, Griffin DK, et al. Artificial oocyte activation with calcium ionophore does not cause a widespread increase in chromosome segregation errors in the second meiotic division of the oocyte. *Fertil Steril* 2016;105:807–814.e2.

37. Vanden Meerschaut F, D'Haeseleer E, Gysels H, et al. Neonatal and neurodevelopmental outcome of children aged 3–10 years born following assisted oocyte activation. *Reprod Biomed Online* 2014;28:54–63.

38. D'haeseleer E, Vanden Meerschaut F, Bettens K, et al. Language development of children born following intracytoplasmic sperm injection (ICSI) combined with assisted oocyte activation (AOA). *Int J Lang Commun Disorders* 2014;49:702–709.

39. Kim JW, Kim SD, Yang SH, et al. Successful pregnancy after SrCl2 oocyte activation in couples with repeated low fertilization rates following calcium ionophore treatment. *Syst Biol Reprod Med* 2014;60:177–182.

40. Yanagida K, Morozumi K, Katayose H, Hayashi S, Sato A. Successful pregnancy after ICSI with strontium oocyte activation in low rates of fertilization. *Reprod Biomed Online* 2006;13:801–806.

41. Kashir J, Nomikos M, Lai FA, Swann K. Sperm-induced Ca2+ release during egg activation in mammals. *Biochem Biophys Res Commun* 2014;450:1204–1211.

42. Nomikos M, Kashir J, Swann K, Lai FA. Sperm PLCzeta: from structure to Ca2+ oscillations, egg activation and therapeutic potential. *FEBS Lett* 2013;587:3609–3616.

43. Sanusi R, Yu Y, Nomikos M, Lai FA, Swann K. Rescue of failed oocyte activation after ICSI in a mouse model of male factor infertility by recombinant phospholipase Czeta. *Mol Hum Reprod* 2015;21:783–791.

44. Lu Q, Zhao Y, Gao X, et al. Combination of calcium ionophore A23187 with puromycin salvages human unfertilized oocytes after ICSI. *Eur J Obstet Gynecol Reprod Biol* 2006;126:72–76.

Chapter 12

Sperm Cryopreservation

Rakesh Sharma, Kruyanshi Master, and Ashok Agarwal

12.1 Introduction

Approximately 30–40 percent of infertility cases represent male factor infertility. In the majority of these cases, patients may opt to freeze their sperm for later use for procreation. Spermatozoa are ideal to cryopreserve because (1) they are the smallest human cells; (2) they have a relatively small volume; (3) a large surface area; (4) they contain very little cytoplasm; (5) less total intracellular water compared to other cells; and (6) they exist individually, allowing effective dehydration. Cryopreservation of spermatozoa is the best option available for having a biological child for these patients [1]. It involves freezing of sperm at extremely low temperatures using liquid nitrogen (LN_2). This process is carried out in the presence of cryoprotectants. Cryprotectants play a critical role in protecting sperm during freezing [2]. In the absence of cryoprotectant spermatozoa can be damaged because of the swelling of the plasma membrane as water expands during freezing, causing acrosomal leakage and breakdown [3]. Glycerol has been used as an effective primary cryoprotectant for freezing spermatozoa [2]. The function of glycerol is to remove or reduce the water content and help minimize intracellular ice formation during freezing. Osmotic equilibrium is reached as the cryoprotectant penetrates the cell and displaces the intracellular water and the sperm returns to almost its original volume. There are a number of factors that may influence and induce abnormal changes in spermatozoa as a result of cryopreservation. These include failure to maintain the optimum temperature and use of diluents that might have negative effects on sperm quality, including reduced semen parameters such as vitality and motility and increased sperm DNA fragmentation [4].

Physicians recommend preservation of gametes especially for adults and young adolescents diagnosed with cancer before they start treatment for cancer. These treatments interfere with the normal functioning of the gametes as well as the process of gametogenesis [5]. To ensure high success rates of the assisted reproduction via sperm cryopreservation, it is necessary to understand the physiology and cryobiology of the sperm. Unlike embryos, sperm cells are smaller in size and have a larger surface area. These characteristics help them to maintain viscosity and the glass transition temperature prevents their cytosol from cryodamage. The role of cytosol is to provide protection from lipid peroxidation and DNA fragmentation [3]. Cooling of sperm cells at lower temperatures ceases all physiological processes and extends their life span [6].

12.2 Sperm Cryopreservation

Cryopreservation is the process of stabilizing the cells at low temperatures (cryogenic temperature) by applying the principles of cryobiology [5]. Freezing of sperm cells for extended periods is possible by arresting their metabolic processes. This can be achieved by storing these cells at $-196\,°C$ in LN_2 [7]. At such a low temperature, the cells dehydrate as a result of water loss due to the formation of ice crystals. The energy of the cells to carry out physiological cycles is reduced. Hence, it becomes easier to store them for longer periods of time [8]. The addition of a cryoprotectant is usually accompanied by a reduction in temperature. As the cooling process continues and the temperature reaches $-5\,°C$ to $-15\,°C$, extracellular ice formation occurs. This induces the development of the extracellular solid phase. The freezing point of water can be reduced to $-42\,°C$ by preventing the process of nucleation – that is, interaction between water droplets to form ice crystals. During the process of cryopreservation, the solutions are cooled below their freezing point without a change in their phase from liquid to solid. This phenomenon is termed supercooling. The formation of ice crystals during this process can be avoided by rapidly reducing the temperature [6]. This starts with forming an ice nucleus in the extracellular space. Solutes are excluded from the ice formed, which increases the concentration of solutes outside the cell. This causes solutes to enter the cell through the plasma membrane and causes them to lose intracellular water, resulting in cell dehydration. During the freezing process, sufficient time should be allowed for sperm cell dehydration and osmotic equilibration. Very slow cooling causes dehydration of the cell while very fast cooling might result in intracellular ice formation. Hence, temperature plays a crucial role here and needs to be controlled accurately [9].

In contrast, when the cells are thawed, the process is reversed. There is a continuous influx of water in the cell, which causes the cells to swell. After a certain period, the cells bursts because of the disruption of the cell membrane. This damage caused by cryopreservation is called cryodamage [2]. The thawing process is as important as the freezing process. The cells should be allowed to restart their physiological activities. Rapid warming can cause heat shock to the cells and damage the cell membrane. Usually 37 °C is used, and higher temperatures are not recommended due to risks associated with cell damage [5]. Cells that have been frozen slowly should also be warmed slowly during thawing, while cells that were frozen rapidly should be thawed rapidly [8]. Although glycerol is a widely used cryoprotectant, it might have negative effects on sperm when added at higher concentrations. The toxicity of glycerol is noted above the concentration of 6%vol./vol. In addition, glycerol also has direct osmotic effects. It tends to cross the plasma membrane comparatively slower than water. For these reasons, addition and removal of glycerol changes the volume of the cell. If the change in volume crosses the osmotic tolerance level of the cell, it causes shrinking or swelling of the cells [6].

12.3 Indications for Sperm Cryopreservation

There are several indications for sperm cryopreservation, including the following:

1. **Cancer**: Men diagnosed with malignant cancer, including testicular cancer, Hodgkin's and non-Hodgkin's lymphoma, leukemia, prostate cancer, and many other types of cancer, prior to radiation therapy for the treatment of cancer [10,11].
2. **Surgery**: Physicians recommend freezing of spermatozoa before undergoing surgeries for vasectomy, vasectomy reversal, or ejaculation failure. Patients with other medical conditions, including varicocele, spinal cord injury, and infections from Zika virus, hepatitis B, or HIV, are also recommended to preserve their fertility [12].
3. **Obstructive or nonobstructive azoospermia**: Sperm are absent in the semen of patients suffering from azoospermia, which may be obstructive or nonobstructive. Sperm cryopreservation is a relevant option for them to preserve fertility [3].
4. **Male factor infertility**: When the infertility is caused due to problems in the male while the female has no abnormal parameters, it is recommended to preserve a semen sample to avoid sterility in a later phase [3].
5. **Autologous or donor sperm cryopreservation**: *Autologous sperm banking* or *client depositor* refers to the individual who preserves spermatozoa for future use with his partner, while a sperm donor is an individual who is serving as a surrogate father for an infertile couple or single female. He may be a directed or anonymous donor. It is necessary for all donors to undergo clinical assessment before sperm donation to avoid infections [6,10].
6. **Occupational**: Occupations with higher exposure to chemicals such as phthalates, pesticides, polychlorinated biphenyls, etc. might affect the fertility in men by increasing oxidative stress and reducing semen parameters. It is recommended to preserve fertility in such cases [12].
7. **Traveling husband/military assignments**: In these cases, it becomes difficult to time intercourse with the process of ovulation. Thus, it is necessary to preserve the semen sample from the husband for future use through assisted reproduction [12].
8. **Gender reassignment**: Approximately three times more individuals opt for male-to-female gender reassignment as compared to female-to-male. These individuals can preserve their sperm before going through gender reassignment and achieve parenthood in the future [10].

12.4 Techniques of Sperm Cryopreservation

12.4.1 Slow Freezing

The principle for this protocol is the formation of ice crystals from extracellular water [13]. This differentiates the two phases: ice crystals formed from

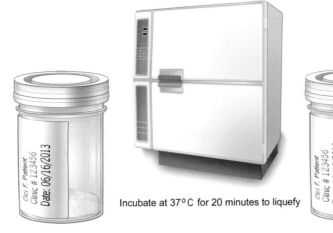

Incubate at 37°C for 20 minutes to liquefy

Figure 12.1 Incubator set at 37 °C and semen sample collected for liquefaction.

extracellular water and water in the liquid phase. The liquid phase consists of cryoprotectants, salts, and sugars [6]. The sperm cells are cooled progressively in several steps over 2–4 hours. This can be carried out manually or with a semi-programmable freezer [5]. The loss of water during this process increases the osmolality of the solution. This causes the cell membrane to shrink. In the andrology laboratory, the commonly used cryoprotectant is modified TES, TRIS and egg yolk buffer (TEST-yolk buffer). The TEST-yolk buffer is an excellent extender that helps maintain sperm viability. Addition of egg yolk helps maintain sperm viability during cryostorage TES, TRIS improves membrane fluidity. Egg yolk-free buffers have also been introduced to avoid potential allergenic reactions and reduce exposure to animal-derived products. Zwitterion buffers also help in the recovery of motile sperm due to their ability to bind free hydrogen and hydroxyl ions in the surrounding medium and to aid in the dehydration process. TEST-yolk buffer contains glycerol. Glycerol has a role in lowering the concentration of salts at an extracellular level by increasing the level of unfrozen water. This decreases the osmotic effects. TEST-yolk consists of low-density lipoproteins which are responsible for protecting the sperm membrane [6]. Sperm suspensions are diluted 1:1 vol./vol. with TEST-yolk buffer, resulting in a final glycerol concentration in the frozen sample of 6 percent. The freezing medium consist of TEST-yolk, glycerol, and gentamicin [14].

In the slow-freezing technique, after complete liquefaction, the freezing medium (TEST-yolk buffer) is added dropwise to the liquefied semen by addition of 25 percent of the semen volume four times, with

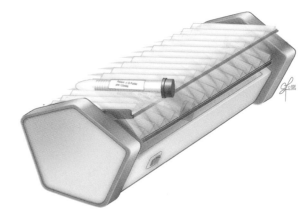

Figure 12.2 Mixing of the semen sample and TEST-yolk on a test tube rocker for 5 min.

5-min interval of slow mixing until a 1:1 sample–medium ratio is achieved [15]. The sample is transferred into the cryovials and frozen at –20 °C for 8 min followed by exposure to the liquid nitrogen vapors at –80 °C (Figures 12.1–12.9). After 2 h of incubation in the vapors, it is preserved in LN_2 at –196 °C [14]. For thawing, the sample is removed from the LN_2 and warmed either slowly at room temperature for 30–40 min or rapidly at 37 °C for 290 min. The conventional slow-freezing protocol performed manually or automated can cause physical and chemical damage to the sperm cell [13].

12.4.2 Rapid Freezing

In the rapid-freezing protocol (less than 15 min), the sample is directly exposed to the nitrogen vapors at –80 °C [5,16]. It is mixed with the cryoprotectant in a

101

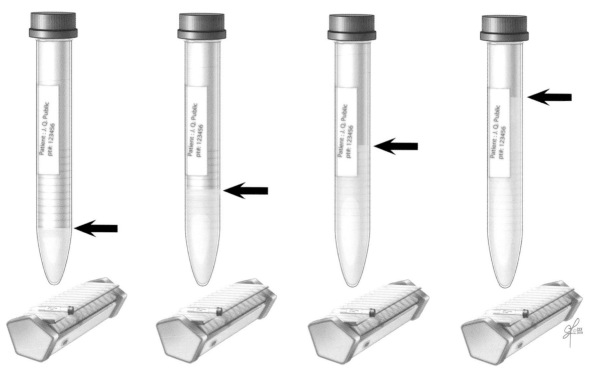

Figure 12.3 Step-wise addition of TEST-yolk equal to one-quarter volume of buffer to patient sample to give a final 1:1 volume.

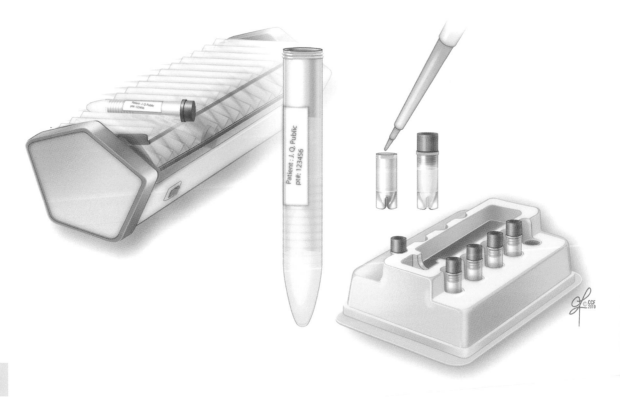

Figure 12.4 Distribution of cryodiluted sample into cryovials using a sterile serological pipette.

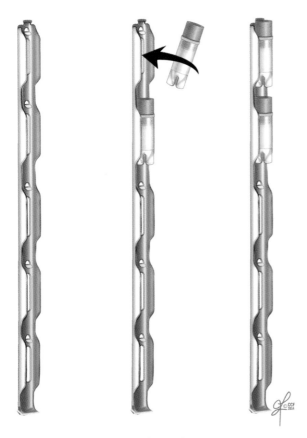

Figure 12.5 Correct loading of cryovials into cryocanes.

dropwise manner and incubated at 4 °C for 10 min. The straws are first placed at a distance of 15–20 cm from the level of the LN_2 for 15 min for vapor exposure, and later immersed in liquid nitrogen at –196 °C [5,17]. Rapid freezing is not used widely because of its low success rate and reproducibility [5]. Controlling the variation in temperature is also difficult [5]. This difficulty can be reduced by using automated programmable freezers, which are easy to use while handling the specimens at different temperatures [17]. The samples are loaded on a cryoplate and placed in the freezer. Automated systems frequently use a cooling rate of –0.5 °C /min from room temperature to –5 °C and a freezing rate of –10 °C/min from –5 °C to –80 °C or –90 °C, followed by immersion in LN_2 [17].

12.4.3 Home Sperm Banking

Home sperm banking is a novel approach for collecting the semen specimen at home. For many patients, collection of a semen specimen is a challenge because

of various factors such as discomfort and stress. Sperm banking facilities are not available in many cities and patients may have to travel from distant places to a sperm banking facility. This may also cause emotional trauma and anxiety. The home sperm banking process is a novel approach for such men that helps overcome the issues related to privacy and anxiety. The NextGen kit is a novel, specially designed kit developed by the Cleveland Clinic Andrology Center for sperm collection and transport (Figure 12.10) [18]. The kit is composed of a collection cup and transportation media, ice sleeves, foam inserts, ice packs, Styrofoam packing box, and the outer box (Figure 12.11). Sample collection and shipping instructions are included in the kit. On receipt of the kit, patients are instructed to place the collection cup, ice packs, freezing sleeve, and refrigeration media in a freezer for at least 12 hours. On the day of collection, before collecting the semen, the refrigeration medium and collection cup are removed from the freezer and allowed to thaw at room temperature for 60 min. The semen sample is deposited by masturbation only, avoiding the use of lubricating gels. After sample collection, the entire content of the refrigeration media (5.0 ml) is added to the collection cup, the cup is sealed securely and gently swirled to mix the contents. The cup is then placed in the kit, along with ice bricks, which are placed on the outside of the foam layers. Finally, the kit is sealed and shipped overnight.

After receiving the sperm sample with the kit, the cryopreservation protocol is carried out as per the slow cryopreservation technique [14]. The effects of overnight transport of the semen specimen on sperm motility using the home sperm banking kit have been examined. Prefreeze and postthaw sperm motility, total motile sperm, and percentage cryosurvival rates were compared between samples collected from infertile men on-site at the Andrology Center ($n = 10$) and samples collected from infertile patients at home (off-site; $n = 9$), and shipped by NextGen to the laboratory (Figure 12.12). A second group ($n = 17$) consisted of 10 semen samples from cancer patients collected on-site, which were compared with seven semen samples from cancer patients shipped by the NextGen [18]. In the infertile men, percentage cryosurvival rates were similar with NextGen compared with those of on-site collection (53.14 ± 28.9 vs 61.90 ± 20.46 percent; $p = 0.51$). Similarly, in the cancer patients, all four parameters were comparable

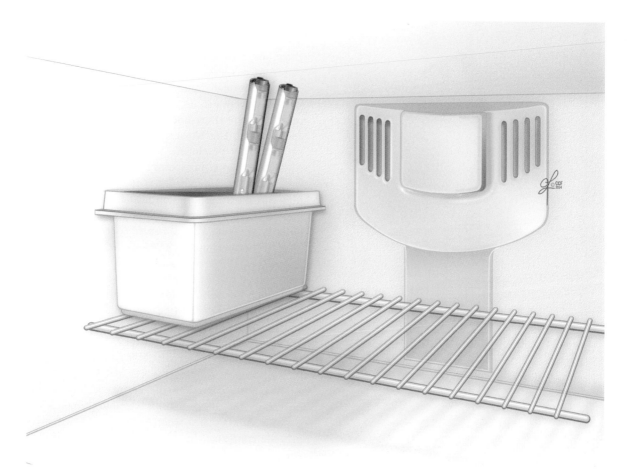

Figure 12.6 Cryovials placed in a cryocane and covered with cryosleeve placed upright in −20 °C freezer for 8 min.

between the on-site and NextGen collections. Cryosurvival rates were also similar between NextGen compared with those of on-site collection (52.71 ± 20.37 vs 58.90 ± 22.68 percent; $p = 0.46$) (Figure 12.13). Cancer patients can bank sperm as effectively as men banking for infertility reasons using the NextGen kit [18].

12.4.4 Sperm Vitrification

Sperm vitrification is an emerging technique for improving reproductive outcomes [4]. The first successful live birth of a human by the vitrification process was documented by researchers at the State University of Iowa in 1953 [19]. Sperm vitrification involves solidification of the specimen at ultralow temperature by elevating its viscosity with a high cooling rate of 15 000–30 000 °C/min [13]. Cooling

cells at such ultracool temperatures creates a glass-like appearance without formation of ice crystals [9,13]. The glass formation occurs efficiently when the cryoprotectant composing the vitrification solution includes the combination of dimethyl sulfoxide, which is a strong glass former, and ethylene glycol, acetamide, and formamide, which are weak glass formers [13].

The vitrification process with cryoprotective agent (CPA) requires exposing the cells to high concentrations of cryoprotectants at room temperature. The sperm wash media for vitrification contains 5% HSA (human serum albumin) and sucrose. Vitrification is not effective with permeable cryoprotectants [20] as this increases the osmolarity [21] and causes human sperm cells to suffer from osmotic shock when exposed to the hypertonic environment. This results in morphological defects

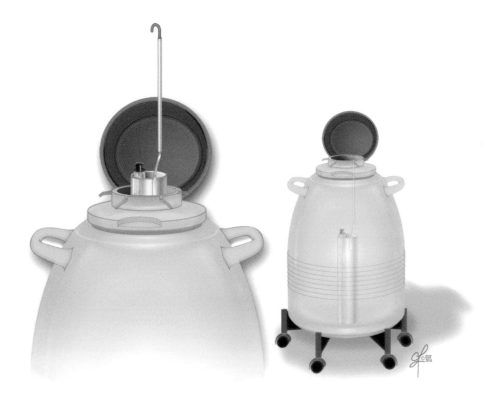

Figure 12.7 Proper loading of cryocanes with cryovials upright into the cryotank canister.

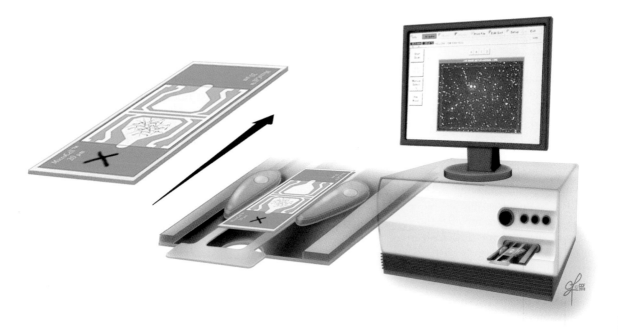

Figure 12.8 Loading of the sperm counting chamber into the load chamber of CASA.

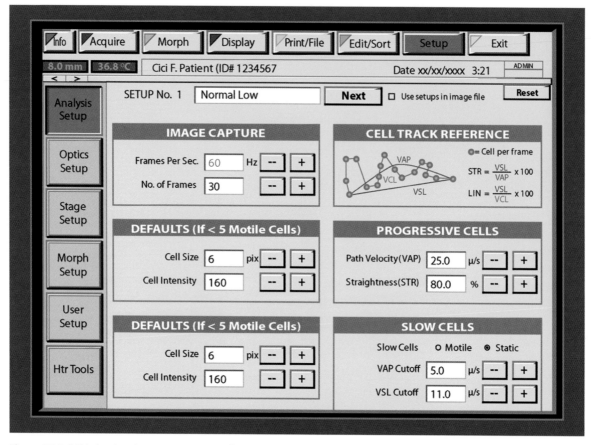

Figure 12.9 CASA showing the screen view setting for sperm motion parameters.

such as coiled tails [20]. This problem can be solved by using isomolar vitrification media which uses nonpermeable cryoprotectants [21]. The sperm suspension is transferred to the cryovial. The cryovial is then placed at the bottom of the cryocane and is exposed to the liquid nitrogen tank [13]. This technique is efficient in maintaining the motility and DNA integrity. It results in higher fertilization and pregnancy rates during the ART procedure compared to the slow-freezing technique. A study conducted on 33 semen samples from humans showed the same outcomes for slow freezing and vitrification [22]. Vitrification is fast, easier, and cost-effective. It has no deleterious effects on sperm quality because of its low toxicity. Sperm vitrification has been performed successfully with and without CPA, but has failed to demonstrate superiority over the conventional sperm-freezing method [4]. In one study, results of conventional slow freezing

and vitrification of 105 human semen samples demonstrated that slow freezing yields better sperm motility and vitality. In contrast to this, vitrification showed better results for sperm morphology [23]. Li et al., in their systematic review, concluded that vitrification is a superior technique compared to conventional slow freezing [24]. They reviewed 2428 studies and showed that total motility and progressive motility of post-thaw semen sample were well preserved by vitrification as compared to conventional slow freezing. However, it is important to note that these results varied on the protocol and the sample size [24].

A new technique called cryoprotectant-free vitrification has been introduced. It is carried out in the absence of cryoprotectants. Vitrification results of 35 human semen samples using the cryoprotectant-free approach showed that high membrane potential and low DNA damage were observed in samples. On

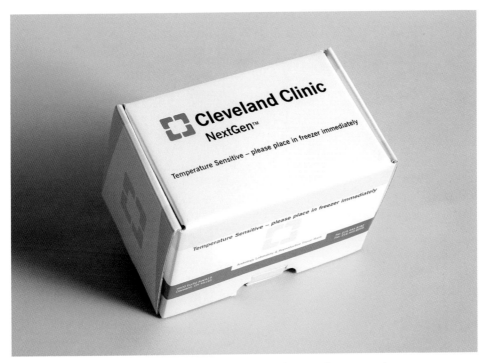

Figure 12.10 View of the NextGen kit optimized for overnight shipping of semen samples.

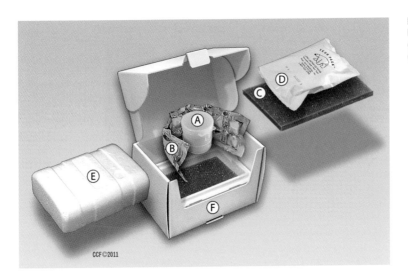

Figure 12.11 Components of the NextGen kit: refrigeration media and (A) collection cup, (B) cooling sleeve, (C) foam insert, (D) ice pack, (E) ice brick, and (F) NextGen box.

the contrary, another study failed to show significant differences in postthaw motility between conventional slow freezing and cryoprotectant-free vitrification [25]. This study was further supported by Aizpurua et al. [26]. This approach yields a greater number of live sperm and maintains the acrosome with reduced DNA fragmentation. Sucrose yields better results in the absence of cryoprotectants. Use of sucrose during vitrification has been correlated with better results in postthaw motility. The plasma membrane and acrosome integrity are also maintained [27].

Sucrose is a sugar and acts like a solute with high viscosity. The increased viscosity during vitrification makes it easy for the cells to achieve a glassy state [13]. Sperm have been shown to be particularly sensitive to

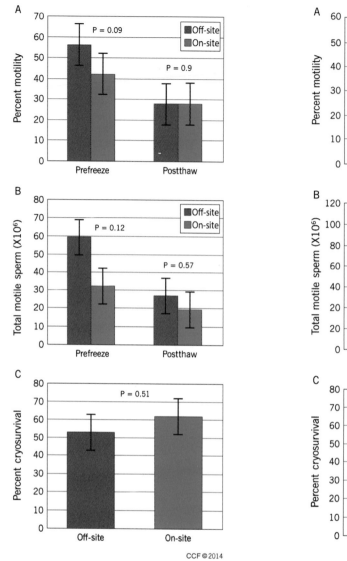

Figure 12.12 Semen samples from off-site and on-site groups of infertile patients showing differences between (A) prefreeze and postthaw percent motility; (B) prefreeze and postthaw total motile sperm; and (C) percent cryosurvival ($n = 7$ off-site and $n = 10$ on-site collections).

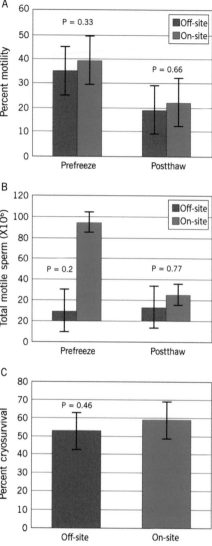

Figure 12.13 Semen samples from off-site and on-site groups of cancer patients showing differences in (A) prefreeze and postthaw percent motility; (B) prefreeze and postthaw total motile sperm; and (C) percent cryosurvival ($n = 7$ off-site; $n = 10$ on-site collections).

exposure to high concentrations of CPAs used routinely in oocyte and embryo vitrification [28,29]. The sperm suspension is directly exposed to the LN_2; however, the non-penetrating cryoprotectants inhibit the flow of water outside the sperm cells and thereby it may cause osmotic damage [13]. In addition to freezing, there is a need for extreme care during the process of thawing. The velocity of thawing plays a challenging role in the cryosurvival rate of

spermatozoa [6]. Despite high-speed freezing of spermatozoa prefreeze, the thawing velocity should be high as well. The reason for this is that the water in the sperm cells must move from the glassy state to the liquid phase. This process should occur without forming ice crystals. Sperm samples show higher motility when thawed at 42 °C [30]. Vitrification of neat ejaculates is associated with several effects on sperm parameters and DNA integrity, suggesting that seminal plasma does not have the same protective effects during sperm vitrification [31].

12.5 Sperm Storage Techniques

Before proceeding with ART, it is recommended to store the sperm cells. The process of cryopreservation damages sperm health on some levels. As a result, the quality of the sperm is reduced in terms of motility [16]. To reduce the amount of damage caused to spermatozoa, it is recommended to store them for only a short interval [32].

In cases of infertility with obstructive and nonobstructive azoospermia, sperm are surgically retrieved and patients are recommended to cryopreserve their samples [3]. Cryopreserving spermatozoa after surgery through the slow-freezing protocol results in an approximately 1 percent recovery rate. Among all the ART procedures, sperm recovery for intracytoplasmic sperm injection (ICSI) is noted to be difficult [33]. There are several methods to cryopreserve spermatozoa, including biological and nonbiological methods [16].

12.5.1 Sperm Storage Inside Zona Pellucida

When the spermatozoa are few in number, they can be stored in the empty zona of human or animals. The process of storing the sperm in zona is critical and requires the stripping of the oocytes. The sperm are aspirated using the ICSI pipette and then transferred to the empty zona [34]. Small holes are created using laser-assisted techniques in the zona membrane to allow the sperm to enter. In the case of the large-sized holes, there are chances for the sperm to leak out and the DNA of the host might enter the oocyte. Small-sized holes may result in entrapped DNA, which causes it to adhere to the sperm. Following the insertion of sperm into the zona, they are frozen using slow freezing. This process has shown a significant improvement in sperm recovery during postthaw [16].

12.5.2 Volvox Globator Spheres

This method is based on the use of an algae named *Volvox globator*. These algae have spherical colonies. Sperm cells are mixed with the cryoprotectants and introduced into the spheres. This process is followed by slow freezing of the spermatozoa. The success rate of this process is noted to be 100 percent [16]. However, the Food and Drug Administration (FDA) restricts the use of this method as the sperm are exposed to algae [1].

12.5.3 Straws and Pipette

The sperm sample can be stored using straws. These straws are distinguished into many types, including open, mini, and open pulled. The open pulled straws use capillary action to help protect samples from mechanical damage. They are highly recommended for the process of vitrification. However, there is a high risk of contamination as the system is open [35]. Mini straws, which are smaller in size, are used when the volume of the sample is comparatively lower. The sample is loaded inside with cryprotectants and the ends of this straw are closed. The disadvantage of this type of straws is that the sperm might stick to the walls [15].

12.5.4 Preserving Spermatozoa Using Microdroplets

The sperm sample, along with cryoprotectants, is rapidly cooled in the presence of dry ice. This process forms microdroplets. These microdroplets are exposed to LN_2 at $-196\ °C$. This method has resulted in six clinical pregnancies (33 percent) [36].

12.5.5 Cryoloop

A study was conducted by Schuster et al. in which they froze the spermatozoa using slow-freezing and ultra-rapid-freezing techniques [16]. The cryoloop method uses a nylon loop that traps the low-volume sample by capillary action [37]. The recovery rate obtained by this process is up to 73 percent. The disadvantage of this process is that it contains a higher risk of contamination because of its open system [38].

12.5.6 Cryotop Method

The cryotop method is an open system. This method is used for individual sperm or a low number of sperm. Sperm cells are transferred to the cryotop strip using the ICSI pipette. It is placed at 4 cm distance from the surface of the LN_2 for 2 min following direct exposure to the LN_2 [13].

12.5.7 Cell Sleeper Method

This method is a closed nonbiological system that consist of a cryovial, which is used as a container. A tray is placed in the cryovial, which can be sealed by a screw cap and mounted on a cryocane, just like a regular cryovial. Approximately 2 µl of spermatozoa droplets prepared by swim-up are transferred on the sleeper cell tray with the help of the ICSI pipette and a micromanipulator. The tray is placed in the cryovial and cooled in LN$_2$ vapors for 2.5 min, followed by immersion in LN$_2$. Sleeper cells have been extremely efficient for cryopreserving small numbers and single sperm [13,39].

12.6 Freezing Spermatozoa

As discussed earlier, cryopreserving spermatozoa at extremely low temperature might cause damage to the DNA and adversely affect the semen parameters, especially motility. In addition to this, the process of freezing and thawing can be detrimental to sperm health [40]. There are several thawing techniques used, including thawing the semen specimen at room temperature for a period of 10 minutes and incubating it at 37 °C for more than 10 minutes. Samples can also be thawed in a water bath at 37 °C for 10 minutes or only thawed at room temperature for 15 min [5].

12.6.1 Cryopreservation of Surgically Retrieved Spermatozoa
12.6.1.1 Testicular Spermatozoa

In male infertility cases such as obstructive and nonobstructive azoospermia, the use of testicular spermatozoa is preferable [41]. The absence of spermatozoa in the ejaculate is the primary reason for retrieving them from the testis. A study by Friedler et al. showed that when the spermatozoa were extracted from the testis and cryopreserved, there was no significant difference observed in the quality of spermatozoa parameters such as fertilization rate, embryo quality, and implantation rate [42]. These results were based on ICSI cycles that compared fresh and cryopreserved spermatozoa retrieved from the testis. The retrieval process for testicular spermatozoa includes open testicular biopsy and testicular sperm aspiration (TESA), and micro-testicular sperm extraction (micro-TESE) [41,43]. Micro-TESE, in comparison with TESE, has a higher retrieval rate [44]. Similar results were obtained in patients diagnosed with obstructive azoospermia [45]. Testicular sperm can be retrieved and cryopreserved for further use [41].

12.6.1.2 Epididymal Spermatozoa

The retrieval of epididymal spermatozoa can be done with either MESA (microsurgical epididymal sperm aspiration) or PESA (percutaneous epididymal sperm aspiration) and is performed on the patients with an obstruction at a site near to the epididymis. In contrast to PESA, sperm retrieval is higher with MESA. These spermatozoa are mature and motile, and thus the sperm selection process becomes easier for ART procedures [41,45].

12.7 Freezing of a Single or Low Number of Spermatozoa

Some patients suffering from nonobstructive azoospermia may have an extremely low number of spermatozoa and hence the sperm retrieval rate in these patients is comparatively lower than for patients with obstructive azoospermia. As a result, cryopreserving a single or a few spermatozoa is a cumbersome process. Single sperm can be cryopreserved by vitrification using sleeper cells or cryotop, both of which are non-biological closed systems [46]. In most cases, for a successful pregnancy the storage techniques of empty zona or cryoloop have also been used [34,37,41,46].

12.8 Fresh vs Frozen Epididymal Spermatozoa

Studies have compared the results of ICSI with fresh semen samples and cryopreserved samples. A study by Tournaye et al. reports that the rate of pregnancy in the ICSI cycle was comparable between fresh and frozen spermatozoa from the epididymis [47]. The study consisted of 53 ICSI cycles with 40 cycles of fresh spermatozoa and 13 cycles of a frozen sample. This study was further supported by the study of Cayan et al., which showed that there was no significant difference between fertility rates with fresh and frozen samples [48]. Opposing this study, Shibahara et al. showed that there is a significant difference between the fertility rate of fresh and frozen epididymal samples [49]. Investigators have shown that the implantation rate can be higher with fresh sperm samples, and that it is more relevant in the case of obstructive than nonobstructive azoospermia [17].

12.9 Fresh vs Frozen Ejaculated Spermatozoa

The two major studies showing the results of ejaculated spermatozoa include one by Kuczynski et al., which consisted of 118 ICSI cycles with fresh spermatozoa and 122 ICSI cycles with frozen spermatozoa

[50]. The study showed no significant difference in the results of the cycles. The authors also state that the rate of pregnancy is significantly higher in ICSI with human samples as compared to other species.

The other study, by Ragni et al., consisted of 79 ICSI cycles that were performed on fresh and frozen samples. They reported no significant differences [51]. In contrast to this, a sample with low sperm motility showed that the fertilization rate with the fresh sample is higher compared to that of a frozen sample. This finding supported the hypothesis that the freezing–thawing process can cause damage to the sperm health and decrease its quality [52].

12.9.1 Detrimental Effects of Freezing on DNA Integrity

Despite the fact that sperm cells are comparatively less susceptible to cryodamage due to low hydration and high membrane fluidity, they may have some detrimental changes [5]. It is noteworthy that semen cryopreservation increases the oxidative stress in sperm cells. Evidence suggests that freezing triggers caspase activity. This requires caspase inhibitors to be added to the medium. Addition of caspase inhibitors maintains motility, both prefreeze and postthaw [12]. In normal conditions, sperm requires healthy DNA, acrosomal reaction, and high motility in order to fertilize an egg. These features of sperm should be preserved even after the postthaw period for successful fertilization during the ART procedure [53]. The amount of reactive oxygen species produced during cryopreservation may also reduce motility and viability, and cause DNA damage by increasing sperm DNA fragmentation. Reports also show changes in the proteome due to cryopreservation. This, in turn, reduces the fertility potential of spermatozoa [17]. Sperm motility is more susceptible to the damage caused by cryopreservation i.e motility is reduced up to 50 percent postthaw [13]. On the other hand, the damage caused to DNA integrity may result in genetic defects [54].

Some studies report significant changes in the DNA integrity after cryopreservation [5]. Contradicting these studies, reports also show no significant damage to the DNA integrity postthaw (Table 12.1). These differences may be attributed to differences in methodology, cryoprotectants used, and the tests used to analyze the integrity of the DNA [5]. In contrast, the study by Donnelly

et al. shows that there was a significant improvement in the DNA integrity of postthaw. This can be because of the presence of high antioxidant levels in seminal plasma [61]. Evidence shows that cryopreservation damages the mitochondrial membrane potential but does not have any adverse impact on DNA integrity. In addition to this, the study by Donnelly et al. also states that sperm DNA from infertile men is more susceptible to cryodamage compared to that from fertile men. Postthaw, there was a significant decrease in DNA integrity of samples from infertile men, while there was no change in the DNA integrity of fertile men [61]. Another study, by Zribi et al., reported that despite the increase in reactive oxygen species (ROS) production during cryopreservation, there is no association between DNA integrity and oxidation. They stated that DNA fragmentation during cryopreservation is not caused by oxidative stress, but by other pathways involving changes in DNA repairing enzymes [65]. However, this hypothesis was rejected by Thomson et al., who reported that DNA fragmentation is a result of an increase in oxidative stress [64]. Certain antioxidants, such as genistein, are found to have lipid peroxidation and SDF-reducing properties. There is increased caspase activity, which can be caused by the cryodamage to the sperm DNA [67]. Based on the literature, the results of DNA damage associated with cryopreservation remains controversial [5].

12.10 Pitfalls and Challenges in Sperm Cryopreservation

There are studies reporting the risk of contamination caused by the leakage of samples in the LN_2. Guidelines are in place for practicing sperm cryopreservation which are helpful in preventing the risks associated with cryopreservation [53]. Cryopreservation of semen samples results in reduced semen parameters such as viability and sperm motility. It is also associated with increased ROS, which causes oxidative stress [17]. Not only sperm motility is affected; cryopreservation can also impair sperm morphology [13]. Sperm damage occurs postthaw, when it is exposed to higher temperatures after long-term storage [17]. Sperm cryopreservation also affects acrosome activity. Studies show that cryopreservation results in a decrease in acrosome activity and acrosome cap, and this is responsible for reduced

Table 12.1 Cryopreservation and its effects on DNA integrity

Cryopreservation method	Sample size	Test to evaluate DNA integrity	Sperm DNA damage induced	Ref.
Equilibration at 37 °C, freezing in liquid nitrogen vapors and storage in liquid nitrogen at −196 °C	19	SCSA+ acridine orange staining	Yes	[55]
Computerized slow freezing + liquid nitrogen vapors	59	Acridine orange staining	Yes	[56]
Equilibration at 37 °C, freezing in liquid nitrogen vapors and storage in liquid nitrogen at −196 °C	19	Acridine orange staining	Yes	[57]
Freezing in liquid nitrogen vapors + computerized programmable freezer	50	Acridine orange staining	Yes	[58]
Freezing in liquid nitrogen vapors	20	Acridine orange staining	Yes	[59]
Freezing with static-phase vapor cooling procedure	196 normozoospermic ($n = 30$); infertile ($n = 166$)	Comet assay	Yes; semen from fertile men more resistant to freezing damage	[60]
Equilibration at 37 °C, freezing in liquid nitrogen vapors and storage in liquid nitrogen at −196 °C	57 fertile ($n = 17$) infertile ($n = 40$)	Comet assay	Yes; semen from fertile men more resistant to freezing damage	[61]
Equilibration at 37 °C, freezing in liquid nitrogen vapors and storage in liquid nitrogen at −196 °C	40	Comet assay	Yes	[61]
Equilibration at 37 °C, freezing in liquid nitrogen vapors and storage in liquid nitrogen at −196 °C	44	Comet assay + acridine orange staining	Yes; morphologically abnormal sperm less resistant to freezing damage	[62]
Freezer at −20 °C, freezing in liquid nitrogen vapors and storage in liquid nitrogen at −196 °C	77	TUNEL assay	Yes	[63]
Programmable freezer	60	TUNEL assay	Yes	[64]
Samples frozen with and without cryoprotectant by slow, controlled-rate method using programmable freezer	320	TUNEL assay	Yes	[64]
Equilibration at 37 °C, freezing in liquid nitrogen vapors and storage in liquid nitrogen at −196 °C	15	TUNEL assay	Yes	[65]
Conventional technique	53 fertile ($n = 20$) infertile ($n = 33$)	Immunoperoxidase detection of digoxigenin-labeled genomic DNA	No	[66]

Table 12.1 (*cont.*)

Cryopreservation method	Sample size	Test to evaluate DNA integrity	Sperm DNA damage induced	Ref.
Freezing in liquid nitrogen vapor	21 control (n = 9) obstructive Azoospermia (*n* = 12)	COMET assay	No	[67]
Programmable slow freezing + vitrification	18	COMET assay	No	[28]
Equilibration at 37 °C, freezing in liquid nitrogen vapor at −80 °C, then storage in liquid nitrogen at −196 °C	21	TUNEL assay + annexin V	No	[68]
Freezing at −20 °C, freezing in liquid nitrogen vapor at −100 °C, then storage in liquid nitrogen at −196 °C	84	TUNEL assay + flow cytometric kit for apoptosis	No	[69]

sperm penetration [13]. Moreover, preserving spermatozoa in LN_2 is a safety hazard. The cryopreservation of spermatozoa is not only time consuming, but also expensive [17].

There is an increase in the damage caused by the cryoprotectants; they might induce some toxic effects when added in high concentrations. This causes changes in the mitochondria by inducing osmotic changes. If the concentration of cryoprotectants are not maintained, it can cause excessive dehydration and ice formation [13]. Freezing of spermatozoa also involves ethical issues. The number of offspring that can be given birth by a single donor is the most common ethical issue due to the unintended blood relation of a donor to the child. Also unresolved is the question of discarding the sperm sample or using it for research in the case that the funding period expires or the couple has a successful pregnancy [10].

12.11 Future Directions

There should be increased awareness among physicians, oncologists, and also patients regarding the importance of cryopreserving sperm for ART procedures [70]. Sperm cryopreservation causes reduced sperm parameters such as motility and viability. Thus, there should be increased use of advanced techniques such as vitrification. Also, the use of open

system carriers might cause cross-contamination. Hence, better options should be considered for storing spermatozoa [16]. Vitrification can also be done using the sleeper cell technique, which preserves a smaller number of sperm. This is preferable as the system is closed and there is a reduced risk of contamination [16].

12.12 Conclusion

Sperm cryopreservation by slow freezing is the most widely used technique for preserving spermatozoa for cancer patients, before treatment for malignant diseases, vasectomy, traveling husbands, or gender reassignment. Sperm cryopreservation is an important component of fertility management, and its successful application affects the reproductive outcome of ART. Patients who do not have access to sperm cryopreservation facilities have the option of freezing their sperm utilizing the NextGen kit. Sperm vitrification is another option available for freezing low sperm numbers of surgically retrieved sperm. Vitrification of sperm means less acrosomal or DNA damage while maintaining sperm motility. The effects of cryopreservation on cells are well documented; the effects on sperm DNA integrity are unclear. Therefore, utmost care should be exercised to provide the maximum protection to the male gamete using techniques aimed at minimizing sperm DNA fragmentation and improving sperm cryosurvival. Although there are several disadvantages of sperm cryopreservation, it is the only option for a man to preserve his fertility and father his biological child.

References

1. AbdelHafez F, Bedaiwy M, El-Nashar SA, Sabanegh E, Desai N. Techniques for cryopreservation of individual or small numbers of human spermatozoa: a systematic review. *Hum Reprod Update* 2008;15:153–164.

2. Holt W. Basic aspects of frozen storage of semen. *Anim Reprod Sci* 2000;62(1–3):3–22.

3. Hezavehei M, Sharafi M, Kouchesfahani HM, et al. Sperm cryopreservation: a review on current molecular cryobiology and advanced approaches. *Reprod Biomed Online* 2018;37 (3):327–339.

4. Agha-Rahimi A, Khalili M, Nottola S, Miglietta S, Moradi A. Cryoprotectant-free vitrification of human spermatozoa in new artificial seminal fluid. *Andrology* 2016;4(6):1037–1044.

5. Di Santo M, Tarozzi N, Nadalini M, Borini A. Human sperm cryopreservation: update on techniques, effect on DNA integrity, and implications for ART. *Adv Urol* 2012;2012: 854837.

6. Mocé E, Fajardo AJ, Graham JK. Human sperm cryopreservation. *EMJ* 2016;1(1):86–91.

7. Hammerstedt RH, Graham JK, Nolan JP. Cryopreservation of mammalian sperm: what we ask them to survive. *J Androl* 1990;11 (1):73–88.

8. Mazur P. Freezing of living cells: mechanisms and implications. *Am J Physiol Cell Physiol* 1984;247(3): C125–C142.

9. Day JG, Harding KC, Nadarajan J, Benson EE. *Cryopreservation: Molecular Biomethods Handbook*. Humuna Press, Totowa, NJ, 2008.

10. Rozati H, Handley T, Jayasena C. Process and pitfalls of sperm cryopreservation. *J Clin Med* 2017;6(9):89.

11. Medrano JV, Del Mar Andrés M, García S, et al. Basic and clinical approaches for fertility preservation and restoration in cancer patients. *Trends Biotechnol* 2018;36(2):199–215.

12. Gupta S, Agarwal A, Sharma R, Ahmady A. Sperm banking via cryopreservation. In: RizkBotros RMB, Aziz N, Agarwal A, Sabanegh E (eds.) *Medical and Surgical Management of Male Infertility*. Jaypee Brothers, New Delhi, 2014, pp. 234–243.

13. Kagalwala S. Sperm vitrification. In Allahabadia G, Kuwayama M, Gandhi G (eds.) *Vitrification in Assisted Reproduction: A User's Manual*. Springer, New Delhi, 2015, pp. 31–42.

14. Agarwal A, Gupta S, Sharma R. Cryopreservation of client depositor semen. In: Agarwal A, Gupta S, Sharma R (eds.) *Andrological Evaluation of Male Infertility: A Laboratory Guide*. Springer, Cham, 2016, pp. 113–133.

15. Agarwal A, Tvrda E. Slow freezing of human sperm. In: Nagy Zsolt P, Vargheses A, Agarwal A (eds.) *Cryopreservation of Mammalian Gametes and Embryos: Methods and Protocols*. Springer Science + Business Media, New York, 2017, pp. 67–78.

16. Sharma R, Kattoor AJ, Ghulmiyyah J, Agarwal A. Effect of sperm storage and selection techniques on sperm parameters. *Syst Biol Reprod Med* 2015;61 (1):1–12.

17. Gupta S, Sharma R, Agarwal A. The process of sperm cryopreservation, thawing and washing techniques. In: Majoub A, Agarwal A (eds.) *The Complete Guide to Male Fertility Preservation*. Springer, Cham, 2018, pp. 183–204.

18. Agarwal A, Sharma R, Gupta S, Sharma R. NextGen® home sperm banking kit: outcomes of offsite vs onsite collection—preliminary findings. *Urology* 2015;85(6):1339–1346.

19. Bunge R, Sherman J. Fertilizing capacity of frozen human spermatozoa. *Nature* 1953;172 (4382):767–768.

20. Oldenhof HM. Gojowsky S, Wang S, et al. Osmotic stress and membrane phase changes during freezing of stallion sperm: mode of action of cryoprotective agents. *Biol Reprod* 2013;88(3):68.

21. Isachenko V, Maettner R, Petrunkina A, et al. Cryoprotectant-free vitrification of human spermatozoa in large (up to 0.5 mL) volume: a novel technology. *Clin Lab* 2011;57(9–10):643–650.

22. Mohamed MSA. Slow cryopreservation is not superior to vitrification in human spermatozoa; an experimental controlled study. *Iranian J Reprod Med* 2015;13(10):633–644.

23. Le MT, Nguyen TTT, Nguyen TT, et al. Cryopreservation of human spermatozoa by vitrification versus conventional rapid freezing: effects on motility, viability, morphology and cellular defects. *Eur J Obstet Gynecol Reprod Biol* 2019;234:14–20.

24. Li YX, Zhou L, LV MQ, et al. Vitrification and conventional freezing methods in sperm cryopreservation: a systematic review and meta-analysis. *Eur J Obstet Gynecol Reprod Biol* 2019;233:84–92.

25. Slabbert M, Du Plessis S, Huyser C. Large volume cryoprotectant-free vitrification: an alternative to conventional cryopreservation for

human spermatozoa. *Andrologia* 2015;47(5):594–599.

26. Aizpurua J, Medrano L, Enciso M, et al. New permeable cryoprotectant-free vitrification method for native human sperm. *Hum Reprod* 2017;32 (10):2007–2015.

27. Isachenko E, Isachenko V, Katkov II, Dessole S, Nawroth F. Vitrification of mammalian spermatozoa in the absence of cryoprotectants: from past practical difficulties to present success. *Reprod Biomed Online* 2003;6(2):191–200.

28. Isachenko E, Isachenko V, Katkov II et al. DNA integrity and motility of human spermatozoa after standard slow freezing versus cryoprotectants-free vitrification. *Hum Reprod* 2004;19:932–939.

29. Isachenko V, Isachenko E, Katkov II et al. Cryoprotectant-free cryopreservation of human spermatozoa by vitrification and freezing in vapor: effect of motility, DNA integrity, and fertilization ability. *Biol Reprod* 2004;71:1167–1173.

30. Mansilla MA, Merino O, Risopatron J, et al. High temperature is essential for preserved human sperm function during the devitrification process. *Andrologia* 2016;48:111–113.

31. Khalili MA, Adib M, Halvaei I, Nabi A. Vitrification of neat semen alters sperm parameters and DNA integrity. *Urol J* 2014;11 (2):1465–1470.

32. Riel JM, Yamauchi Y, Huang TT, Grove J, Ward MA. Short-term storage of human spermatozoa in electrolyte-free medium without freezing maintains sperm chromatin integrity better than cryopreservation. *Biol Reprod* 2011;85(3):536–547.

33. Podsiadly BT, Woolcott RJ, Stanger JD, Stevenson K. Pregnancy resulting from intracytoplasmic injection of cryopreserved spermatozoa

recovered from testicular biopsy. *Hum Reprod* 1996;11 (6):1306–1308.

34. Cohen J, Garrisi GJ, Congedo-Ferrara TA, et al. Cryopreservation of single human spermatozoa. *Hum Reprod* 1997;12(5):994–1001.

35. Isachenko V. Clean technique for cryoprotectant-free vitrification of human spermatozoa. *RBM Online* 2005;10(3):350–354.

36. Gil-Salom MJ, Romero C, Rubio A, Remohı RJ, Pellicer A. Intracytoplasmic sperm injection with cryopreserved testicular spermatozoa. *Mol Cell Endocrinol* 2000;169(1-2):15–19.

37. Lane M, Bavister BD, Lyons EA, Forest KT. Containerless vitrification of mammalian oocytes and embryos. *Nat Biotechnol* 1999;17 (12):1234–1236.

38. Schuster TG, Keller LM, Dunn RL, Ohl DA, Smith GD. Ultra-rapid freezing of very low numbers of sperm using cryoloops. *Hum Reprod* 2003;18 (4):788–795.

39. Endo Y, Fujii Y, Shintani K, et al. Simple vitrification for small numbers of human spermatozoa. *Reprod Biomed Online* 2012;24:301–307.

40. Royere D, Hamamah S, Nicolle J, Lansac J. Chromatin alterations induced by freeze–thawing influence the fertilizing ability of human sperm. *Int J Androl* 1991;14(5):328–332.

41. Gangrade BK. Cryopreservation of testicular and epididymal sperm: techniques and clinical outcomes of assisted conception. *Clinics* 2013;68:131–140.

42. Friedler S, Strassburger D, Raziel A, et al. Intracytoplasmic injection of fresh and cryopreserved testicular spermatozoa in patients with nonobstructive azoospermia: a comparative study. *Fertil Steril* 1997;68(5):892–897.

43. Moskovtsev S, Lulat A, Librach C. *Cryopreservation of Human Spermatozoa by Vitrification vs. Slow Freezing: Canadian Experience.* Intech Open, London, 2012.

44. Schlegel PN. Testicular sperm extraction: microdissection improves sperm yield with minimal tissue excision. *Hum Reprod* 1999;14:131–135.

45. Esteves SC; Miyaoka R, Agarwal A. Sperm retrieval techniques for assisted reproduction. *Int Braz J Urol* 2011; 37(5): 570–583.

46. Desai N, Blackmon H, Goldfarb J. Single sperm cryopreservation on cryoloops: an alternative to hamster zona for cryopreservation of individual spermatozoa. *Fertil Steril* 2003;80:55–56.

47. Tournaye H, Merdad T, Silber S, et al. No differences in outcome after intracytoplasmic sperm injection with fresh or with frozen–thawed epididymal spermatozoa. *Hum Reprod* 1999;14(1):90–95.

48. Cayan S, Lee D, Conaghan J, et al. A comparison of ICSI outcomes with fresh and cryopreserved epididymal spermatozoa from the same couples. *Hum Reprod* 2001;16(3):495–499.

49. Shibahara H, Hamada Y, Hasegawa A, et al. Correlation between the motility of frozen-thawed epididymal spermatozoa and the outcome of intracytoplasmic sperm injection. *Int J Androl* 1999;22(5):324–328.

50. Kuczynski W, Dhont M, Grygoruk C, et al. The outcome of intracytoplasmic injection of fresh and cryopreserved ejaculated spermatozoa: a prospective randomized study. *Hum Reprod* 2001;16(10):2109–2113.

51. Ragni G, Caccamo AM, Dalla Serra A, Guercilena S. Computerized slow-staged freezing of semen from men with testicular tumors or Hodgkin's disease preserves sperm better

than standard vapor freezing. *Fertil Steril* 1990;53(6):1072–1075.

52. Borges E Jr, Rossi LM, Locambo de Freitas CV, et al. Fertilization and pregnancy outcome after intracytoplasmic injection with fresh or cryopreserved ejaculated spermatozoa. *Fertil Steril* 2007;87(2):316–320.

53. Gupta S, Sekhon LH, Agarwal A. Sperm banking: when, why, and how? In: Sabanegh ES Jr. (ed.) *Male Infertility. Current Clinical Urology: Male Infertility: Problems and Solutions.* Springer, Cham, 2011, pp. 107–118.

54. Kliesch S, Kamischke A, Cooper TG, Nieschlag E. Cryopreservation of human spermatozoa. In: *Andrology*, Springer, Cham, 2010, pp. 505–520.

55. Spanò M, Cordelli E, Leter G, et al. Nuclear chromatin variations in human spermatozoa undergoing swim-up and cryopreservation evaluated by the flow cytometric sperm chromatin structure assay. *Mol Hum Reprod* 1999;5(1):29–37.

56. Hammadeh ME, Dehn C, Hippach Zeginiadou M, et al. Comparison between computerized slow-stage and static liquid nitrogen vapour freezing methods with respect to the deleterious effect on chromatin and morphology of spermatozoa from fertile and subfertile men. *Int J Androl* 2001;24(2):66–72.

57. Gandini l, Lombardo F, Lenzi A, Spanò M, Dondero F. Cryopreservation and sperm DNA integrity. *Cell Tissue Banking* 2006;7(2):91–98.

58. Petyim S, Choavaratana R. Cryodamage on sperm chromatin according to different freezing methods, assessed by AO test. *J Med Assoc Thailand* 2006;89(3):306–313.

59. Ngamwuttiwong T, Kunathikom S. Evaluation of cryoinjury of sperm chromatin according to liquid nitrogen vapour method (I). *J Med Assoc Thailand* 2007;90(2):224–228.

60. Ahmad L, Jalali S, Shami SA, et al. Effects of cryopreservation on sperm DNA integrity in normospermic and four categories of infertile males. *Syst Biol Reprod Med* 2010;56(1):74–83.

61. Donnelly ET, McClure N, Lewis SE. Cryopreservation of human semen and prepared sperm: effects on motility parameters and DNA integrity. *Fertil Steril* 2001;76(5):892–900.

62. Kalthur G, Adiga SK, Upadhya D, Rao S, Kumar P. Effect of cryopreservation on sperm DNA integrity in patients with teratospermia. *Fertil Steril* 2008;89(6):1723–1727.

63. de Paula TS, Bertolla RP, Spaine DM, et al. Effect of cryopreservation on sperm apoptotic deoxyribonucleic acid fragmentation in patients with oligozoospermia. *Fertil Steril* 2006;86(3):597–600.

64. Thomson LK, Fleming SD, Aitken RJ, et al. Cryopreservation-induced human sperm DNA damage is predominantly mediated by oxidative stress rather than apoptosis. *Hum Reprod* 2009;24(9):2061–2070.

65. Zribi N, Chakroun NF, El Euch H, et al. Effects of cryopreservation on human sperm deoxyribonucleic acid integrity. *Fertil Steril* 2010;93(1):159–166.

66. Høst E, Lindenberg S, Kahn JA, Christensen F. DNA strand breaks in human sperm cells: a comparison between men with normal and oligozoospermic sperm samples. *Acta Obstet Gynecol Scand* 1999;78(4):336–339.

67. Steele EK, McClure N, Lewis SEM. Comparison of the effects of two methods of cryopreservation on testicular sperm DNA. *Fertil Steril* 2000;74(3):450–453.

68. Duru NK, Morshedi MS, Schuffner A, Oehninger S. Cryopreservation-thawing of fractionated human spermatozoa is associated with membrane phosphatidylserine externalization and not DNA fragmentation. *J Androl* 2001;22(4):646–651.

69. Paasch U, Sharma RK, Gupta AK, et al. Cryopreservation and thawing is associated with varying extent of activation of apoptotic machinery in subsets of ejaculated human spermatozoa. *Biol Reprod* 2004;71(6):1828–1837.

70. Varghese AC, Nandi P, Mahfouz R, Athayde KS, Agarwal A. *Human Sperm Cryopreservation: Andrology Laboratory Manual.* Jaypee Brothers, New Delhi, 2010, pp. 196–208.

Chapter 13

Future Directives in Sperm Handling for ART

Catalina Barbarosie, Manesh Kumar Panner Selvam, and Ashok Agarwal

13.1 Background

Fertilization is a complex process that takes place when the spermatozoa penetrates and fuses with the oocyte to form a zygote. To make fertilization possible, both gametes must experience a series of preparatory steps. Human spermatozoa develop from a series of multi-step processes from spermatogenesis, spermiogenesis in the male reproductive tract, to capacitation in the female reproductive tract [1].

Approximately 15 percent of couples who engage in unprotected intercourse for more than one year have issues conceiving. Between 20 and 70 percent of these couples experience male infertility factor [2]. A high number of couples with fertility problems resort to assisted reproduction techniques (ARTs). More than 2,500 procedures per one million women were performed in 2015 in the USA [3]. Assisted reproduction techniques include approaches such as intrauterine insemination (IUI), *in vitro* fertilization (IVF), and intracytoplasmic sperm injection (ICSI). The role of sperm selection techniques is to mimic the natural selection process and activate the oocyte. The techniques for sperm handling are very important as they allow for improved ART success. The natural selection of competent sperm for oocyte insemination is bypassed in ICSI. Since IVF and ICSI outcomes are dependent on sperm characteristics, it is important to select a high-quality sperm with good motility, morphology, viability, and DNA integrity [4].

Sperm selection techniques have been developed to handle and select the most capable sperm for oocyte fertilization, and to obtain a healthy offspring. The first sperm selection techniques developed were swim-up and density gradient centrifugation, which select spermatozoa according to mobility and viability. However, these techniques are unable to distinguish spermatozoa with high levels of oxidative stress and poor DNA integrity [5]. Consequently, advanced sperm selection techniques have been developed to overcome these limitations. The advanced techniques test the sperm membrane markers, size, motility, and other characteristics. These techniques separate immature and abnormal spermatozoa and those with low DNA integrity, leukocytes, cell debris, microorganisms, and antisperm antibodies from the seminal plasma [6]. More noninvasive future sperm selection techniques are under development to allow the selection of high-quality cells in real time, for their immediate use in ART [5]. In this chapter we present the current sperm selection methods, as well as the future techniques for sperm handling and selection before ART (Table 13.1).

13.2 Conventional Sperm Processing Techniques

13.2.1 Swim-Up

The swim-up technique selects highly motile and morphologically normal spermatozoa based on their ability to swim out of the seminal plasma into the upper layer containing medium. This technique can be performed using a washed sperm pellet (conventional swim-up) or whole liquefied semen specimen (direct swim-up) [7]. The conventional swim-up method consists of several centrifugation steps, which results in the generation of reactive oxygen species (ROS), leading to decreased sperm motility and plasma membrane integrity, increased apoptosis, and DNA fragmentation [8]. The direct swim-up technique was specially developed for oligozoospermic semen samples to overcome the negative impact of centrifugation steps on spermatozoa [8,9]. The migration–sedimentation method was developed for spermatozoa with reduced motility, and the swim-down technique allows selection of highly motile sperm in a downward gradient [9].

The direct swim-up method is cost-effective and the easiest technique for sperm separation by migration. The liquefied semen specimen is placed into round-bottom tubes, followed by stratification with

Table 13.1 List of sperm handling/selection techniques for ART

No.	Technique	Principle/procedure	Advantages	Disadvantages
1 Conventional sperm processing techniques				
1.1	Swim-up technique	• Tests the ability of sperm to swim out of the seminal plasma into the layer containing isotonic sperm wash medium. • Selects highly motile and morphologically normal spermatozoa.	• Cost-effective and easy to perform.	• Generation of reactive oxygen species. • Low recovery rate of sperm.
1.2	Density gradient centrifugation	• Separates motile from nonmotile sperm cells and cellular debris based on their relative density. • Selects highly motile and viable sperm.	• Easy and fast method. • High rate of sperm recovery.	• Risk of obtaining sperm with low DNA integrity and contaminated with endotoxins
2 Advanced sperm processing techniques				
2.1	Magnetic-activated cell sorting	• Separates apoptotic from non-apoptotic sperm cells. • Selects sperm with higher progressive motility, normal morphology, high DNA integrity, and non-disturbed mitochondrial membrane potential.	• Simple, reliable, and noninvasive technique.	• Accidental microbeads can be injected into the oocyte along with the spermatozoa during ICSI. • Should be performed in combination with other semen sample processing technique.
2.2	Microfluidics	• Separates sperm with high motility and normal morphology. • Selects sperm with normal morphology, high chromatin condensation, and high DNA integrity.	• Nontoxic to the sperm. • Low-volume semen samples can be used. • No centrifugation steps are required.	–
2.3	Motile sperm organelle morphology examination	• Assess morphologic characteristics at the subcellular level. • Selects sperm without subcellular morphological abnormalities.	• Sperm are assessed in real time. • Analyzed at higher magnification and low sperm suspension sample can be used.	• Expensive and labor-intensive technique.
2.4	Flow cytometry	• Sorts sperm according to their physical, chemical, or fluorescent markers. • Assess important sperm parameters such as sperm count, viability, acrosomal reaction, mitochondrial membrane potential, and DNA integrity and capacitation status.	• Differentiates between X- and Y-sperm carrying chromosomes. • Recovers non-apoptotic spermatozoa from a sperm suspension.	• Requires skilled technologist. • High-speed sorting can damage the plasma membrane and affects viability and motility of the spermatozoa.

Table 13.1 (*cont.*)

No.	Technique	Principle/procedure	Advantages	Disadvantages
2.5	Electrophoretic sperm selection	• Differentiates mature sperm from immature and dysfunctional sperm, as well as from leukocytes based on the size and charge.	–	• Currently not being used in ART facilities.
2.6	Zeta potential	• Selects mature sperm that has more negative charge compared to cellular debris. • Selects high-quality mature spermatozoa with normal morphology, high DNA integrity, and chromatin condensation, able to undergo hyperactivation.	• Fresh and cryopreserved semen samples can be used.	• Low sperm recovery rate.
2.7	Hyaluronic acid binding assay	• Selects mature sperm with hyaluronic acid (HA) binding sites, which are markers for high DNA integrity.	• Selected spermatozoa have higher viability, motility, and morphology, lower DNA fragmentation levels, lower rate of chromosomal aneuploidies and apoptotic markers.	–
3 Future sperm selection techniques				
3.1	Raman spectrometry	• Assesses the DNA structure and sites of damage. • Evaluates the mitochondrial membrane potential and motility status of human spermatozoa.	• Noninvasive and nondestructive technique.	• Sensible to room temperature changes. • Time-consuming steps involved in sperm specimen preparation.
3.2	Interferometric phase microscopy	• Quantitatively images sperm cells.	• Stain-free technique.	• Immobilization step may harm sperm cells.
3.3	Confocal light absorption and scattering spectroscopic microscopy	• Gives deeper-tissue images and provides high specific contrast images. • Allows visualization of individual organelles in living cells at a scale of 100 nm.	• Label-free technique and does not damage the cell structure or DNA molecule.	• Requires more standardization. • Time-consuming steps involved in sperm specimen preparation.
3.4	Proteomic analysis and peptide-based selection	• Detects damage and binds to fragmented DNA.	• Identifies single-stranded DNA and single- and double-stranded DNA breaks.	• Requires sperm membrane removal.

sperm wash medium. The tubes with the samples are placed at a 45° angle in the incubator for 1 h at 37 °C, followed by aspiration of viable sperm from the upper layer [9,10]. The viable sperm swims up through the medium, while the nonmotile sperm remains at the bottom of the tube (Figure 13.1). Finally, sperm analysis is done to determine whether the sperm parameters such as count and motility are sufficient for IUI [11]. Ideally, a total motile sperm count of 5×10^6 is utilized for IUI [12]. Youglai et al. reported

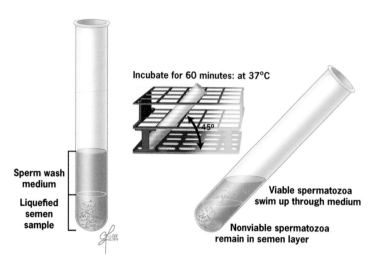

Figure 13.1 Swim-up procedure. The upper layer contains sperm wash medium and the bottom one the liquefied semen sample. After incubation, the motile spermatozoa will swim up into the upper layer, and the nonviable sperm, leukocytes, and cell debris will remain at the bottom of the tube.

that there was no difference between the conventional and direct swim-up methods with respect to sperm DNA damage and ability of recovered spermatozoa to fertilize the oocyte [13].

The swim-up technique is fast and cost-effective. The selected sperm are highly motile, with improved motion characteristics compared to unselected ones [14]. Furthermore, sperm selected with swim-up before freezing (cryopreservation) have higher post-thaw motility, acrosome integrity, and ability to undergo acrosome reaction [14]. However, one of the major limitations of this technique is the low rate of sperm recovery (5–10 percent) [9].

13.2.2 Density Gradient Centrifugation

The density gradient centrifugation technique is considered to be the gold standard approach for semen selection [15]. This method separates motile from nonmotile sperm cells and cellular debris according on their density. For this, the spermatozoa cross a gradient made with colloidal silicon and stop at a specific density layer according to their isopycnic point [8]. Live and motile spermatozoa have different density compared to immature or dead spermatozoa. Live and motile spermatozoa have slightly higher density of at least 1.10 g/ml, and settle in the bottom layer (80 percent). Abnormal nonmotile sperm have a slightly lower density of 1.06–1.09 g/ml, and they are retained in the middle layer (40 percent) [16]. The cell debris and leukocytes are collected at the interphase between the seminal plasma and the 40 percent upper phase [16]. There are several approaches to this technique, which include continuous and discontinuous density gradient methods [9].

The two-layer discontinuous density gradient technique is easy to perform and consists of adding the lower phase (80 percent), layering the upper phase (40 percent), followed by the liquefied semen specimen in a graduated conical centrifuge tube. The tube is centrifuged for 20 minutes at 1600 rpm (Figure 13.2) [9]. After centrifugation, the supernatant consisting of seminal plasma, abnormal nonmotile sperm, and both interphases are completely removed and the sperm pellet at the bottom of the tube is resuspended with 2 ml of sperm wash medium. This is further centrifuged for 7 min at 1600 rpm. Again, the supernatant is discarded and the washed sperm pellet is resuspended in a final volume of 0.5 ml of sperm wash medium. The density gradient centrifugation is an easy and fast method. In contrast with the swim-up method, it has a higher rate of sperm recovery, and is the preferred method for semen specimens with low sperm concentration or abnormal morphology or motility. However, there is a higher risk of obtaining spermatozoa with low DNA integrity and contaminated with endotoxins [9].

13.3 Advanced Sperm Processing Techniques

13.3.1 Magnetic-Activated Cell Sorting

The magnetic-activated cell sorting (MACS) technique uses annexin V-conjugated paramagnetic microbeads to differentiate and eliminate apoptotic cells from a sperm suspension. In apoptotic spermatozoa, the phospholipid phosphatidylserine is translocated from the inner leaflet to the outer leaflet of the

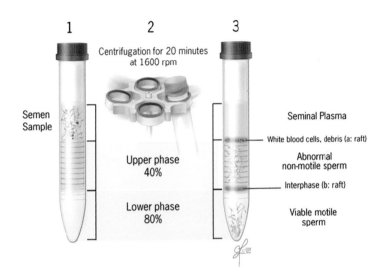

1   2   3

Centrifugation for 20 minutes at 1600 rpm

Semen Sample

Upper phase 40%

Lower phase 80%

Seminal Plasma

White blood cells, debris (a: raft)

Abnormal non-motile sperm

Interphase (b: raft)

Viable motile sperm

Figure 13.2 Density gradient centrifugation procedure. The lower phase is followed by the upper phase and semen sample. After centrifugation, the viable mature spermatozoa will be present in the bottom layer. The abnormal nonmotile and seminal plasma will be in the upper and seminal plasma layers, respectively.

plasma membrane. Consequently, the phosphatidylserine is considered an apoptotic marker. This technique is based on the fact that annexin V protein has high affinity for phosphatidylserine expressed at the outside plasma membrane of apoptotic sperm [5,9].

The liquefied semen specimen is incubated with annexin V-conjugated paramagnetic beads for 15 min at room temperature. During the incubation step, the apoptotic spermatozoa attach to the annexin V-coated microbeads as a result of interaction between phosphatidylserine and annexin V protein. Then, the sperm suspension is passed through the column, which is placed on a stand surrounded by a magnetic field. While the non-apoptotic spermatozoa (annexin V-negative) passes through the magnetic field along with the solution, drop by drop, in the collection tube, the apoptotic (annexin V-positive) spermatozoa are retained in the magnetic field (Figure 13.3). The viable, non-apoptotic (annexin V-negative) sperm collected in the solution can be used for ART [17].

This technique is simple, reliable, and noninvasive. Sperm sorted with MACS have higher progressive motility, normal morphology, high DNA integrity, and non-disturbed mitochondrial membrane potential [5]. This technique alone allows obtaining sperm with lower DNA fragmentation by 30 percent. When MACS is used in combination with density gradient centrifugation, a further relative reduction in sperm DNA fragmentation of 40 percent is obtained [6]. The microbeads used in the MACS technique are considered harmless for sperm cells as

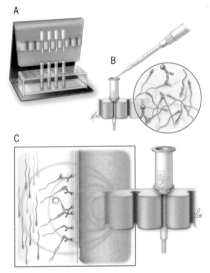

A

B

C

Figure 13.3 (a) MACS stand. (b) After incubation, sperm suspension is placed into a column which is placed on a stand surrounded by a magnetic field. (c) While the non-apoptotic spermatozoa pass through the column into the solution, the apoptotic spermatozoa, attached to the magnetic microbeads, are retained in the magnetic field.

they are composed of microspheres (50 nm in diameter) made up of iron [18]. However, care should be taken that no microbeads are injected into the oocyte along with the spermatozoa during ICSI. As the MACS technique does not eliminate leukocytes and cell debris, it should be performed before or after

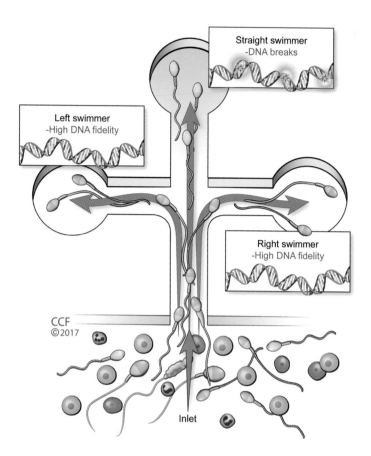

Figure 13.4 Microfluidic device able to select sperm according to their motility capacity. Immotile and immature sperm, leukocytes, and cell debris remain in the inlet compartment. Motile sperm with high levels of DNA damage swim straight. Motile spermatozoa with high DNA integrity swim to the right and left compartments.

other semen sample processing techniques such as swim-up and density gradient centrifugation [6].

13.3.2 Microfluidics

Microfluidics is a relatively new technique introduced in the field of sperm selection. It uses a nontoxic and transparent microchannel made of polydimethylsiloxane (PDMS) silicon polymers that separates sperm with high motility and normal morphology [17]. There are several approaches within this technique. However, the passively microfluidic device had demonstrated better results in selecting motile sperm without the need for centrifugation steps [19].

These devices mimic the female reproductive tract with respect to fluid viscosity and temperature. The dead and nonmotile sperm, leukocytes, and cell debris in the liquefied semen are unable to move and are retained in the inlet. While sperm with DNA breaks swim straight, sperm with high DNA integrity swim to the left and right outlets (Figure 13.4) [17]. This allows the selection of sperm with normal morphology, high

chromatin condensation, and high DNA integrity from a low-volume semen sample (1 ml) [20]. The spermatozoa are collected in a 100 μl final volume of the buffer.

13.3.3 Motile Sperm Organelle Morphology Examination

Motile sperm organelle morphology examination (MSOME) was developed as a sperm selection technique based on morphologic characteristics at the subcellular level (head components, mid-piece, tail region, mitochondria, nucleus chromatin content, presence and size of vacuoles). The spermatozoa are assessed in real time at a high magnification (6300×) using an inverted light microscope equipped with Nomarski optics [21].

This technique allows the visualization of sperm at a higher magnification compared with the one used for routine semen analysis. It makes possible the selection of spermatozoa without subcellular morphological abnormalities [6]. The MSOME protocol involves mixing 1 μl of sperm suspension with 5 μl of human tubal fluid (HTF) (containing 7 percent polyvinylpyr-rolidone solution). The mixture is placed in a glass Petri dish and observed under an inverted light microscope at a high magnification. Then, the images are captured and the morphologically normal sperm can be selected for ICSI. The combination of MSOME and ICSI has been named intracytoplasmic morphologically selected sperm injection (IMSI) [21]. This is a costly, time-consuming, labor-intensive process and requires a skilled technologist to select the best sperm [22,23].

13.3.4 Flow Cytometry

The flow cytometric cell sorting technique is used to differentiate specific cell populations from a sample. This method allows assessing important sperm parameters such as sperm count, viability, acrosomal reaction, mitochondrial membrane potential, DNA integrity, and capacitation status [24]. Specific sub-populations of sperm cells, such as cells with high DNA integrity, high mitochondrial membrane potential, and non-apoptotic cells can be analyzed and sorted according to their physical, chemical, or fluorescent markers [17,24]. Moreover, flow cytometry can differentiate between X- and Y-sperm carrying chromosomes and can be used as a selection technique to reduce the risk of having a child with X- or Y-linked disorders [24].

The sperm cells are washed, diluted, and suspended in appropriate medium, such as modified Tyrode's albumin–lactate–pyruvate (TALP) buffer or binding buffer [17,25]. Next, they are either directly (primary antibodies – fluorescent-conjugated monoclonal antibodies) or indirectly (using secondary conjugated antibodies) labeled with fluorescent probes. The primary antibody recognizes and binds directly to a target antigen, whereas the secondary antibody binds to a primary antibody that is attached to a target antigen. Then, the sperm are passed thorough the flow channel and excited by the laser to generate fluorescence signals. The photomultiplier detects the light scatter and fluorescent signals. The optic system records and amplifies the signals obtained by the photomultiplier tubes. The signals recorded by the machine are converted into data files that can be analyzed using software.

This process allows sorting the sperm based on their emitted fluorescence. Finally, different sperm subpopulations are collected in separate wash media [17,24]. The sorted spermatozoa can be used either for IUI, IVF, or ICSI.

It is considered that sperm sorting using flow cytometry efficiently recovers non-apoptotic spermatozoa from a sperm suspension [17]. However, a recent study by De Geyter et al. reported that removal of DNA-fragmented spermatozoa using flow cytometry did not significantly improve the ICSI outcome compared to the swim-up technique [26]. Also, it should be taken into consideration that the sperm cells pass through the flow system very quickly, and they reach a speed of about 90 km/h when they exit the nozzle at the routine sorting pressure of 50 psi (standard pressure). This can damage the plasma membrane and affects viability and motility of the spermatozoa. Suh et al. demonstrated that lowering the standard pressure from 50 psi to 40 psi can improve the parameters of sorted sperm cells, such as concentration and motility [25].

13.3.5 Electrophoretic Sperm Selection

Plasma membrane of matured spermatozoa with normal morphology contains a high concentration of sialic acid, which induces negative charge to the sperm. The electrophoretic approach allows differentiating mature sperm from immature and dysfunctional sperm, as well as from leukocytes based on the size and charge [17]. Microcell flow and microelectrophoresis are two methods used for electrophoretic sperm selection.

The microcell flow consists of two outer and two inner chambers, separated by a 5-μm pore polycarbonate membrane. The inner chamber consists of an inoculation chamber and a collection compartment. The outer chamber is connected with platinum-coated titanium electrodes [6]. The semen specimen (400 μl) is loaded into the inoculation chamber and allowed to migrate from the negative (cathode) to positive pole (anode) for 5 min at 23 °C, with a constant current of 75 mA and variable voltage of 18–21 V, followed by collection of mature sperm from the collection compartment [27]. The spermatozoa with high negative charge are able to migrate from the cathode to the anode within 5 min because the plasma membrane contains a high concentration of sialic acid. The immature sperm cannot migrate within this time because they contain lower concentrations of sialic acid in the plasma membrane, so carry less negative charge. Larger cells such as leukocytes and immature germ cells are filtered/trapped at the polycarbonate membrane level (Figure 13.5) [17]. This technique allows recovery of sperm of good

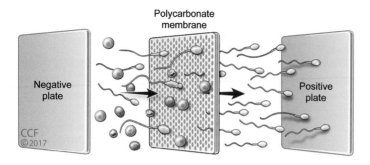

Figure 13.5 Microcell flow device consisting of a polycarbonate membrane able to let highly negative-charged mature spermatozoa migrate from cathode to anode. The leukocytes, immature spermatozoa, and cell debris stop at the polycarbonate membrane level.

quality (motility, normal morphology, and DNA integrity), able to capacitate and bind to the zona pellucida. Furthermore, the selected sperm are free from leukocytes and other contaminants [5,27].

The microelectrophoresis approach differentiates sperm with low levels of DNA damage from abnormal spermatozoa based on electrical charge. The microelectrophoresis consists of an electrophoresis chamber, an egg injection chamber, two bubble restriction chambers, one conductive bridge, and a power pack [28]. After density gradient centrifugation and adjusting sperm concentration at 20×10^6/ml, 10–15 µl of selected sperm is loaded into the electrophoretic buffer at increasing current from 6 mA to 14 mA and variable voltage (30–100 V). The ability of sperm to migrate from cathode to anode is monitored with an inverted microscope, and one spermatozoa is picked up for ICSI [28].

13.3.6 Zeta Potential

The electrical potential at the slipping plane of the sperm cell in suspension, away from the interface, is called sperm zeta potential or electrokinetic potential [5]. The plasma membrane of mature sperm is negatively charged, and it has a zeta potential ranging from –16 mV to –20 mV [5,9]. This technique is based on the fact that mature spermatozoa have a more negative charge than does cellular debris. In addition, mature spermatozoa with zeta potential adhere to surfaces positively charged in a medium without proteins.

Briefly, 100 µl of washed sperm is loaded into a glass tube and mixed with 5 ml of serum-free HEPES-HTF medium. Glass tubes are preferred as they are positively charged (2–4 mV) [29]. The glass tube is placed into a latex glove, rotated two or three times, and withdrawn from the glove. The tube is incubated for 1 min at room temperature. During the incubation, mature spermatozoa with negative zeta potential

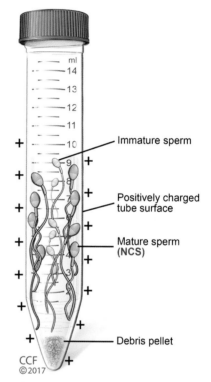

Figure 13.6 Spermatozoa selection based on zeta potential. Mature negatively charged spermatozoa (NCS) bind to the tube's positively charged surface. The immature spermatozoa are unable to bind to the tube's surface and the cell debris gather at the bottom of the tube.

stick to the walls of the tube (Figure 13.6). Then the tube is centrifuged at 300 g for 5 min, which does not change the electric charge in the tube. The supernatant is discarded and 200 µl serum-supplemented HEPES-HTF medium is added to wash the mature sperm adhering to the tube's walls. The addition of serum neutralizes the surface charge by binding to anions and cations in the solution [29]. During all the steps, the tube should be held vertically.

This technique is preferable when compared with the density gradient centrifugation method. The zeta potential technique selects high-quality mature spermatozoa with normal morphology, high DNA integrity, and chromatin condensation, able to undergo hyperactivation [29,30]. Both fresh and cryopreserved semen samples are used as cryopreservation does not affect the zeta potential of the sperm membrane. This technique is also used to select X-bearing sperm as they have higher zeta potential than Y-bearing sperm [5]. The recovery rate of sperm is very low, making this method limited for oligozoospermic samples [6]. More studies are required to determine if zeta potential is a reliable test for clinical application.

13.4 Processing of Banked Sperm for ART

Cryopreservation is the technique used to bank sperm at cryogenic temperatures. It is performed by slow freezing (from room temperature to –196 °C) the semen sample processed mostly using TEST-yolk buffer (TYB). The TYB is a freezing medium that contains tris, sodium citrate, fructose, egg yolk, glycerol, and gentamicin. The samples are kept at –20 °C for 20 min, then maintained at –86 °C for 60 min, and finally stored at –196 °C [31]. To improve the sperm quality, sperm selection techniques can be used both before and after cryopreservation.

Allamaneni et al. compared the postthaw sperm parameters of both swim-up and gradient density centrifugation selected sperm. Sperm selected with gradient density centrifugation had higher post-thaw total motile sperm count ($p = 0.003$), recovery rate ($p = 0.003$), and motility ($p = 0.011$) at 4 h (32.2×10^6/ml, 69.2 and 83 percent, respectively) compared to sperm selected with the swim-up technique (17.6×10^6/ml, 50 and 55 percent, respectively) [32]. Said et al. reported that selection of postthaw sperm using MACS resulted in sperm with impaired motility, whereas better results were noticed when MACS sperm selection was done before the cryopreservation step [33].

Zeta potential may also be a possible technique for the selection of cryopreserved sperm. Postthaw selected sperm using the zeta potential technique had better morphology (62 percent) and intact acrosome (40 percent). Furthermore, sperm necrosis and apoptosis were lower in postthawed selected sperm (12 and 64 percent, respectively). However, the progressive motility decreased by 50 percent. The

recovered sperm can be used for ICSI, as the sperm recovery rate using this technique was only 8–10 percent [34]. The electrophoresis-based selection technique has a recovery rate of 27 percent [35]. The decision in choosing IUI, IVF, or ICSI will depend on the post-cryopreservation sperm concentration.

13.5 Sperm Handling Approach and Outcome in ART

13.5.1 Intrauterine Insemination

Intrauterine insemination is the simplest and most commonly used ART method to help infertile couples conceive. The swim-up technique is recommended for the selection of sperm from normozoospermic infertile cases due to its low recovery rate [14]. The pregnancy rate using swim-up for IUI in couples with unexplained infertility was 11 percent [36]. Intrauterine insemination with selected motile sperm $<0.8 \times 10^6$/ml after swim-up had a pregnancy rate of less than 1 percent per treatment, whereas IUI performed using motile sperm $>0.8 \times 10^6$/ml had a better pregnancy rate (6.9–10.2 percent) [37]. A Cochrane review showed that there is no significant difference in pregnancy rate for couples undergoing IUI between the swim-up and gradient centrifugation techniques (30.5 and 21.5 percent, respectively), and between swim-up and wash followed by centrifugation (22.2 and 38.1 percent, respectively) [38]. The gradient technique is more effective than swim-up for IUI success in couples with unexplained subfertility, with an ongoing pregnancy rate per patient of 26.4 percent [36]. The one-step density gradient and two-step discontinuous density gradient techniques are recommended for normozoospermic semen samples and for couples undergoing IVF or ICSI, but not IUI [7]. Using the gradient centrifugation, the total motile sperm count, recovery rate, and sperm longevity at 2 h were 32.2×10^6/ml, 69.2 percent, and 83 percent, respectively [32].

13.5.2 *In Vitro* Fertilization and Intracytoplasmic Sperm Injection

13.5.2.1 Hyaluronic Acid Binding Assay Outcome

Mature spermatozoa contain hyaluronic acid (HA) binding sites that recognize the HA contained in the cumulus–oophorus–corona radiata complex. The presence of HA binding sites is a marker of mature spermatozoa with high DNA integrity [6]. There are two methods for HA binding: sperm–hyaluronan binding assay and physiological spermatozoa for ICSI (PICSI) [5]. The sperm–hyaluronan binding assay selects functional sperm with high fertilizing potential and is used for both IVF and ICSI [6]. Spermatozoa selected by HA assay have higher viability, motility, and morphology. In addition, they have lower DNA fragmentation levels and lower rates of chromosomal aneuploidies and apoptotic markers [6].

A systematic review reported that sperm selected with HA binding assay had lower DNA fragmentation and the fertilization rate for ICSI was higher in one study. However, the same systematic review presents other studies in which HA binding spermatozoa selected for ICSI improved the embryo quality and cleavage rate, but did not improve the fertilization rate [39]. Additional studies suggest that sperm selection with HA assays results in sperm with lower percentages of chromosome aneuploidies [40], higher DNA integrity, and improved embryo quality [41]. In contrast, other researchers identified no difference regarding the zygote score between sperm bound and unbound to HA [5]. Oehninger and Kotze reported that patients had higher implantation rate compared with control individuals (37.4 vs 30.7 percent) and lower pregnancy loss rate (3.3 vs 15.1 percent) when sperm HA binding efficiency before ICSI was more than 65 percent [42].

13.5.2.2 PICSI Outcome

In order to perform the PICSI technique, washed sperm is placed at the edge of the HA spot on a Petri dish. Then the spermatozoa that bind to the HA are collected and used for ICSI [39]. The PICSI technique was reported to provide better results regarding fertilization rate compared to control ones (79.4 vs 67.7 percent, respectively, $p = 0.02$) [39,43]. Also, lower miscarriage rates were reported with the PICSI technique [6]. In contrast, Avalos-Duran et al. summarized that there was no statistically significant difference between PICSI and ICSI outcomes with respect to embryo quality, pregnancy, implantation, miscarriage, and fertilization rates [44]. A recent report from Miller et al. confirmed that use of the PICSI technique did not improve the live birth rate compared to standard ICSI [45].

13.5.2.3 Microfluidics Outcome

The microfluidic device selects high-quality spermatozoa with normal morphology, high chromatin condensation, and low levels of ROS. The DNA integrity and vitality were improved up to 80 and 89 percent, respectively [17,19]. Furthermore, the use of the microfluidics approach was suggested to be associated with increased likelihood of having euploid embryos (71 percent) [46]. Sperm selected using microfluidic devices have better morphology and higher motility compared with those selected by swim-up or unselected sperm [47]. Yetkinel et al. reported no significant differences in the fertilization (63.6 and 57.4 percent), clinical pregnancy (48.3 and 44.8 percent), and live birth (38.3 and 57.4 percent) rates with sperm selected by microfluidic and conventional swim-up approaches for ICSI in patients with unexplained infertility [48]. Microelectrophoresis can select high negatively charged mature spermatozoa [28]. Newer microfluidic devices have been developed to select spermatozoa according to sperm motility and ability to swim in the direction of a chemoattractant or temperature limit, and to cross streamlines in a laminar fluid stream. However, these devices are currently used for research purposes, and no data related to human ART outcomes has been published [49].

13.5.2.4 MSOME Outcome

Among all the sperm abnormalities identified using the MSOME method, the shape and chromatin content are associated with establishment of pregnancy [21]. The MSOME technique seems to improve the clinical outcomes in patients with previous ICSI failures, leading to a higher pregnancy rate [39]. A meta-analysis compared ICSI and IMSI outcomes, and reported that top-quality embryo rate (41.2 vs 27.7 percent), implantation rate (21.9 vs 10.5 percent), and pregnancy rate (47.6 vs 26.6 percent) were higher, while the miscarriage rate (14.7 vs 29 percent) was lower with IMSI [50]. In contrast, De Vos et al. showed no difference between IMSI and ICSI in relation to clinical pregnancy rate (34.4 vs 36.7 percent) [51]. A recent meta-analysis of randomized studies reported no clinical advantage of IMSI over ICSI regarding live birth and miscarriage rates [52].

13.6 Future Sperm Selection Techniques

13.6.1 Raman Spectrometry

Raman spectrometry is a noninvasive and nondestructive technique that provides information about the biomolecular constituents and chemical composition of a cell [6], such as information about the sperm DNA structure and damage [17]. Raman spectrometry captures the vibration of molecular constituents of the sample to analyze the internal biological structure [53]. This is a powerful tool to assess the DNA structure and sites of damage, and the mitochondrial membrane potential and motility status of human spermatozoa [6].

In general, analysis of sperm is done in real time. It includes washing and smearing the sample on a quartz coverslip, followed by Raman spectrometry detection [54]. However, more studies are warranted to determine whether this technology is harmless for the semen specimen analyzed before using the selected sperm for ICSI. Furthermore, this technique is highly sensitive to room temperature changes and sperm specimen preparation [54].

13.6.2 Interferometric Phase Microscopy

The interferometric phase microscopy is a stain-free technique used to quantitatively image sperm cells. This technique uses only one source of light that is split into two beams. A digital camera superimposes the light that passes through a sample with a reference beam that does not. By combining the two beams, an interferogram is obtained. The interferogram is translated through digital processing into a quantitative phase map [55]. The sperm selected using swim-up is diluted with 5 ml of HTF medium. A volume of 10 μl of the diluted semen sample is placed on a cover glass. The sample is covered by a small cover glass, and sperm are immobilized by heating at 60 °C for 5 min. The immobilized sample is analyzed using an interferometric phase microscope. Reports indicate that the immobilization step does not harm the sperm plasma membrane and sperm morphology, but additional studies should be done to prove this fact [55]. Eravuchira et al. used the standard density gradient centrifugation to separate the spermatozoa before analyzing them with interferometric phase microscopy. The sorted sperm

cells were mixed with HTF medium and centrifuged for 5 min at 400 rcf at room temperature. Then, the sperm were collected and mixed with modified HTF medium. The spermatozoa with 7 percent polyvinylpyrrolidone (PVP) were introduced into a microchamber in a ratio of 1:1. The role of PVP is to increase the viscosity of the solution to provide better visualization of sperm [56].

13.6.3 Confocal Light Absorption and Scattering Spectroscopic Microscopy

Confocal light absorption and scattering spectroscopy (CLASS) works based on two principles: confocal microscopy and light scattering spectroscopy. This technique is able to obtain deeper-tissue images and provide high specific contrast images [5]. The particles beyond the diffraction limit are detected and characterized [57]. It is a label-free technique and does not damage the cell structure or DNA molecule. This tool allows visualizing individual organelles in living cells at a scale on the order of 100 nm. CLASS microscopy can discriminate between two different cell subpopulations (apoptotic and non-apoptotic human bronchial epithelial cells) [57]. This technique could be applied for sperm selection before ART as it does not damage the structure of the sperm cell [17].

13.6.4 Proteomic Analysis and Peptide-Based Selection

Enciso et al. designed a synthetic peptide (DW1) of 21 amino acids that correspond to the human p53 molecule, and labeled it with a terminal dye. The synthetic oligopeptide was able to detect damage and bind to fragmented DNA (Figure 13.7). This peptide identifies single-stranded DNA and single- and double-stranded DNA breaks only after membrane removal. Because this technique involves sperm membrane removal, the analyzed spermatozoa cannot be used for ART procedures [58].

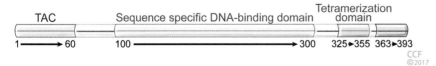

Figure 13.7 Organization of the p53 synthetic protein. It consists of three main domains: TAC, sequence specific DNA-binding, and tetramerization domains.

13.7 Conclusion

Overall, ART outcomes have not improved over the last few decades. Therefore, efforts are needed to improve the available techniques for sperm handling and selection, but also to develop methods that are able to increase the live birth rate after ART. The current techniques do not provide sufficient information to overcome the fertility problems. Also, most of the techniques that test the quality of sperm also damage the cell structure, rendering the spermatozoa unsuitable for ICSI. Therefore, future techniques that diagnose spermatozoa in real time should be applied before undergoing ART techniques.

References

1. Sharma R, Agarwal A. *Spermatogenesis: an overview*. In: Zini A, Ashok A (eds.) *Sperm Chromatin*. Springer, New York, 2011, pp. 19–44.

2. Agarwal A, Mulgund A, Hamada A, Chyatte MR. A unique view on male infertility around the globe. *Reprod Biol Endocrinol* 2015;13 (1):37.

3. Sunderam S, Kissin DM, Crawford SB, et al. Assisted reproductive technology surveillance: United States, 2015. *MMWR Surveill Summ* 2018;67 (3):1–28.

4. Tarozzi N, Nadalini M, Borini A. Effect on sperm DNA quality following sperm selection for ART: new insights. *Adv Exp Med Biol* 2019;1166:169–187.

5. Henkel R. Sperm preparation: state-of-the-art: physiological aspects and application of advanced sperm preparation methods. *Asian J Androl* 2012;14(2):260.

6. Tarozzi N, Nadalini M, Borini A. Effect on sperm DNA quality following sperm selection for ART: new insights. In: Baldi E, Muratori M (eds.) *Genetic Damage in Human Spermatozoa*. Springer, New York, 2019, pp. 169–187.

7. Gangrade BK, Agarwal A. Sperm processing and selection techniques in an IVF/ICSI. In: Varghese AC, Sjoblom P, Jayaprakasan K (eds.), *A Practical Guide to Setting Up an IVF Lab, Embryo Culture Systems and Running the Unit*. JP Medical, London, 2013, pp. 151–159.

8. Muratori M, Tarozzi N, Carpentiero F, et al. Sperm selection with density gradient centrifugation and swim up: effect on DNA fragmentation in viable spermatozoa. *Sci Rep* 2019;9 (1):7492.

9. Beydola T, Sharma RK, Lee W, et al. Sperm preparation and selection techniques. In: Rizk BRMB, Aziz N, Agarwal A, Sanbanegh E (eds.) *Male Infertility Practice*. Jaypee Brothers, New Delhi, 2013, pp. 244–251.

10. Otsuki J, Chuko M, Momma Y, Takahashi K, Nagai Y. A comparison of the swim-up procedure at body and testis temperatures. *J Assist Reprod Genet* 2008;25(8):413–415.

11. Agarwal A, Gupta S, Sharma R. Sperm preparation for intrauterine insemination (IUI) by swim-up method. In: Agarwal A, Gupta S, Sharma R (eds.) *Andrological Evaluation of Male Infertility*. Springer, New York, 2016, pp. 109–112.

12. Dickey RP, Pyrzak R, Lu PY, Taylor SN, Rye PH. Comparison of the sperm quality necessary for successful intrauterine insemination with World Health Organization threshold values for normal sperm. *Fertil Steril* 1999;71(4):684–689.

13. Younglai EV, Holt D, Brown P, Jurisicova A, Casper RF. Sperm swim-up techniques and DNA fragmentation. *Hum Reprod* 2001;16(9):1950–1953.

14. Esteves SC, Sharma RK, Thomas AJ Jr, Agarwal A. Effect of swim-up sperm washing and subsequent capacitation on acrosome status and functional membrane integrity of normal sperm. *Int J Fertil Women Med* 2000;45 (5):335–341.

15. Grunewald S, Paasch U. Sperm processing and selection. In Parekattil SJ, Agarwal A (eds.) *Male Infertility: Contemporary Clinical Approaches, Andrology, ART & Antioxidants*. Springer, New York, 2012, pp. 423–430.

16. Malvezzi H, Sharma R, Agarwal A, Abuzenadah AM, Abu-Elmagd M. Sperm quality after density gradient centrifugation with three commercially available media: a controlled trial. *Reprod Biol Endocrinol* 2014;12(1):121.

17. Agarwal A, Selvam MKP. Advanced sperm processing/selection techniques. In: Zini A, Agarwal A (eds.) *A Clinician's Guide to Sperm DNA and Chromatin Damage*. Springer, New York, 2018, pp. 529–543.

18. Molday RS, Yen SPS, Rembaum A. Application of magnetic microspheres in labelling and separation of cells. *Nature* 1977;268(5619):437–438.

19. Asghar W, Velasco V, Kingsley JL, et al. Selection of functional human sperm with higher DNA integrity and fewer reactive oxygen species. *Adv Healthcare Mater* 2014;3 (10):1671–1679.

20. Nosrati R, Vollmer M, Eamer L, et al. Rapid selection of sperm

with high DNA integrity. *Lab Chip* 2014;14(6):1142–1150.

21. Bartoov B, Berkovitz A, Eltes F, et al. Real-time fine morphology of motile human sperm cells is associated with IVF-ICSI outcome. *J Androl* 2002;23(1): 1–8.

22. Perdrix A, Saïdi R, Ménard JF, et al. Relationship between conventional sperm parameters and motile sperm organelle morphology examination (MSOME). *Int J Androl* 2012;35 (4):491–498.

23. Ebner T, Shebl O, Oppelt P, Mayer RB. Some reflections on intracytoplasmic morphologically selected sperm injection. *Int J Fertil Steril* 2014;8(2):105–112.

24. Mahfouz RZ, Said TM, Agarwal A. The diagnostic and therapeutic applications of flow cytometry in male infertility. *Arch Med Sci* 2009;5(1A):S99–S108.

25. Suh TK, Schenk JL, Seidel GE, Jr., High pressure flow cytometric sorting damages sperm. *Theriogenology* 2005;64 (5):1035–1048.

26. De Geyter C, Gobrecht-Keller U, Ahler A, Fischer M. Removal of DNA-fragmented spermatozoa using flow cytometry and sorting does not improve the outcome of intracytoplasmic sperm injection. *J Assist Reprod Genet* 2019;36 (10):2079–2086.

27. Ainsworth C, Nixon B, Aitken RJ. Development of a novel electrophoretic system for the isolation of human spermatozoa. *Hum Reprod* 2005;20 (8):2261–2270.

28. Simon L, Murphy K, Aston KI, et al. Optimization of microelectrophoresis to select highly negatively charged sperm. *J Assist Reprod Genet* 2016;33 (6):679–688.

29. Chan PJ, Jacobson JD, Corselli JU, Patton WC. A simple zeta method for sperm selection based on

membrane charge. *Fertil Steril* 2006;85(2):481–486.

30. Kheirollahi-Kouhestani M, Razavi S, Tavalaee M, et al. Selection of sperm based on combined density gradient and zeta method may improve ICSI outcome. *Hum Reprod* 2009;24(10):2409–2416.

31. Martins AD, Agarwal A, Henkel R. Sperm cryopreservation. In: Nagy ZP, Varghese A, Agarwal A (eds.) *In Vitro Fertilization*. Springer, New York, 2019, pp. 625–642.

32. Allamaneni SS, Agarwal A, Rama S, et al. Comparative study on density gradients and swim-up preparation techniques utilizing neat and cryopreserved spermatozoa. *Asian J Androl* 2005;7(1):86–92.

33. Said TM, Grunewald S, Paasch U, et al. Effects of magnetic-activated cell sorting on sperm motility and cryosurvival rates. *Fertil Steril* 2005;83(5):1442–1446.

34. Kam TL, Jacobson JD, Patton WC, Corselli JU, Chan PJ. Retention of membrane charge attributes by cryopreserved-thawed sperm and zeta selection. *J Assist Reprod Genet* 2007;24 (9):429–434.

35. Ainsworth C, Nixon B, Jansen RP, Aitken RJ. First recorded pregnancy and normal birth after ICSI using electrophoretically isolated spermatozoa. *Hum Reprod* 2006;22(1):197–200.

36. Karamahmutoglu H, Erdem A, Erdem M, et al. The gradient technique improves success rates in intrauterine insemination cycles of unexplained subfertile couples when compared to swim up technique; a prospective randomized study. *J Assist Reprod Genet* 2014;31 (9):1139–1145.

37. Berg U, Brucker C, Berg FD., Effect of motile sperm count after swim-up on outcome of intrauterine insemination. *Fertil Steril* 1997;67(4):747–750.

38. Boomsma CM, Heineman MJ, Cohlen BJ, Farquhar CM. Semen preparation techniques for intrauterine insemination. *Cochrane Database Syst Rev* 2004;3:CD004507.

39. Said TM Land JA. Effects of advanced selection methods on sperm quality and ART outcome: a systematic review. *Hum Reprod Update* 2011;17(6):719–733.

40. Jakab A, Sakkas D, Delpiano E, et al. Intracytoplasmic sperm injection: a novel selection method for sperm with normal frequency of chromosomal aneuploidies. *Fertil Steril* 2005;84 (6):1665–1673.

41. Parmegiani L, Cognigni GE, Bernardi S, et al. "Physiologic ICSI": hyaluronic acid (HA) favors selection of spermatozoa without DNA fragmentation and with normal nucleus, resulting in improvement of embryo quality. *Fertil Steril* 2010;93(2):598–604.

42. Oehninger SC, Kotze D. Sperm binding to the zona pellucida, hyaluronic acid binding assay, and PICSI. In: Agarwal A, Borges E, Jr., Setti AS (eds.) *Non-Invasive Sperm Selection for In Vitro Fertilization: Novel Concepts and Methods*, Springer, New York, 2015, pp. 59–68.

43. Nasr-Esfahani MH, Razavi S, Vahdati AA, Fathi F, Tavalaee M. Evaluation of sperm selection procedure based on hyaluronic acid binding ability on ICSI outcome. *J Assist Reprod Genet* 2008;25(5):197–203.

44. Avalos-Durán G, Cañedo-Del Ángel AME, Rivero-Murillo J, et al. Physiological ICSI (PICSI) vs. conventional ICSI in couples with male factor: a systematic review. *JBRA Assist Reprod* 2018;22(2):139.

45. Miller D, Pavitt S, Sharma V, et al. Physiological, hyaluronan-selected intracytoplasmic sperm injection for infertility treatment (HABSelect): a parallel, two-

group, randomised trial. *Lancet* 2019;393(10170):416–422.

46. Parrella A, Choi D, Keating D, Rosenwaks Z, Palermo GD. A microfluidic device for selecting the most progressively motile spermatozoa yields a higher rate of euploid embryos. *Fertil Steril* 2018;110(4):e342.

47. Chinnasamy T, Behr B, Demirci U. Microfluidic sperm sorting device for selection of functional human sperm for IUI application. *Fertil Steril* 2016;105(2):e17–e18.

48. Parrella A, Choi D, Keating D, Rosenwaks Z, Palermo GD. Effects of the microfluidic chip technique in sperm selection for intracytoplasmic sperm injection for unexplained infertility: a prospective, randomized controlled trial. *J Assist Reprod Genet* 2019;36(3):403–409.

49. Knowlton SM, Sadasivam M, Tasoglu S. Microfluidics for sperm research. *Trends Biotechnol* 2015;33(4):221–229.

50. Souza Setti A, Ferreira RC, Paes de Almeida Ferreira Braga D, et al. Intracytoplasmic sperm injection outcome versus intracytoplasmic morphologically selected sperm injection outcome: a meta-analysis. *Reprod Biomed Online* 2010;21(4):450–455.

51. De Vos A, Van de Velde H, Bocken G, et al. Does intracytoplasmic morphologically selected sperm injection improve embryo development? A randomized sibling-oocyte study. *Hum Reprod* 2013;28 (3):617–626.

52. Duran-Retamal M, Morris G, Achilli C, et al. Live birth and miscarriage rate following intracytoplasmic morphologically selected sperm injection vs intracytoplasmic sperm injection: an updated systematic review and meta-analysis. *Acta Obstet Gynecol Scand*, 2019;99:24–33.

53. Brauchle E, Schenke-Layland K. Raman spectroscopy in biomedicine–non-invasive in vitro analysis of cells and extracellular matrix components in tissues. *Biotechnol J* 2013;8 (3):288–297.

54. Liu Y, Zhu Y, Li Z. Application of Raman spectroscopy in andrology: non-invasive analysis of tissue and single cell. *Transl Androl Urol* 2014;3(1):125.

55. Mirsky SK, Barnea I, Levi M, Greenspan H, Shaked NT. Automated analysis of individual sperm cells using stain-free interferometric phase microscopy and machine learning. *Cytometry A* 2017;91(9):893–900.

56. Eravuchira PJ, Mirsky SK, Barnea I, et al. Individual sperm selection by microfluidics integrated with interferometric phase microscopy. *Methods* 2018;136:152–159.

57. Itzkan I, Qiu L, Fang H, et al. Confocal light absorption and scattering spectroscopic microscopy monitors organelles in live cells with no exogenous labels. *PNAS* 2007;104 (44):17255–17260.

58. Enciso M, Pieczenik G, Cohen J, Wells D. Development of a novel synthetic oligopeptide for the detection of DNA damage in human spermatozoa. *Hum Reprod* 2012;27(8):2254–2266.

Index

131